Asperger's Ready for Battle.

The 2nd Encounter. No more secrets.

Simon. R. Newell.

Asperger's Ready for Battle.
The 2nd Encounter. No more secrets.
Simon. R. Newell.

ISBN 978-1-909660-64-9

A CIP catalogue record for this book
is available from the British Library

Published 2016 by Tricorn Books
131 High Street, Old Portsmouth
PO1 2HW

www.tricornbooks.co.uk

Printed and bound in UK

Asperger's Ready for Battle.

The 2nd Encounter. No more secrets.

Contents.

Testimonial.

In Response to Book 1 The Plain Truth. By Kevin Kearn. Friend to our family.

Hello Simon,

I thought you might be interested in reading some of my reflections on your first book. I have no real experience of reviewing books so these are simply my impressions and my attempt to highlight those aspects of your ideas that are particularly stimulating.

This is a challenging book in the very best sense of the word 'challenging'. It is not simply a book which can be read and forgotten, or a book which can be read like a novel, although it does contain within it, a good deal of your own story. Your weaving together of the bigger picture with your own personal journey is, in my view, highly effective in keeping the reader focused.

You challenge us, your readers, to seek to understand Asperger's syndrome and, more importantly, to understand and appreciate those who live with it.

To do so you identify a number of 'problems' and 'symptoms' associated with the condition. The list is long 41, and in each example you go beyond identifying the 'problem' to a discussion of how it might be addressed and ameliorated. You explain, from personal experience, that individuals who are considered to have Asperger's are likely to experience some of these 'problems' and experience them to different degrees and in varying intensity. My understanding of this aspect of your argument is that to be an 'aspie' (to adopt one of your favourite 'handles') is not to conform to some kind of standard model; each individual's experience is unique.

It also strikes me that some of the symptoms you identify are common to many of us at various times in our lives.

It follows that Asperger's syndrome is a matter of degree and intensity rather than of a clear distinction between those of us who have Asperger's and those who don't. Your book would have been worth writing for these insights alone.

Your discussion of the anxieties that often arise from social encounters are both moving and informative.

You have captured so well the stresses that can and so often do accompany meeting new people and in sustaining social contacts, and friendships. I am left with the impression that it is these which can provide some of the most difficult situations that people with Asperger's face.

As if this were not enough, you are conscious of the need to try and put people you meet at their ease! This, of course, is a reflection of widespread public ignorance of the condition.

Your view from the inside is so much richer than could ever come from the pen of a 'professional'.

Perhaps your book will contribute to reducing a woeful lack of knowledge and understanding among the general population. Having said that, I know from other fields, that 'raising awareness' is extremely difficult and can often feel fruitless. No one could ever say that you haven't played your part in this enterprise.

At a purely personal level, I very much enjoyed your discussion in chapter 8 of 'Government Issues, Work, Taxpayers'. Your perspectives on these provide another challenge to conventional wisdom (which you term the majority opinion). In my view you hit the nail on the head in arguing that the approach adopted by successive governments - and reinforced in political propaganda - is both narrow and ill-informed.

We live in a society that increasingly appears to function on the assumption that only those activities which result in payment are of any value; anything else is futile. The clear implication is that 'paid work' should be the highest of our personal aspirations and our social objectives.

This, as you argue, reveals a poverty of spirit which

diminishes us as individuals and degrades us as a community.

Once we come to accept that only those human activities which can command a price have any value, we are surely on the road to dismantling the best of our civilisation. It's hard to imagine that the 'Work Capability Assessment' will ever be cited as a major landmark on our road to creating a fair society.

Finally, perhaps among the most attractive feature of your work, is what I can only describe as its intimacy. You explain that your writing style is personal and unconventional but, if I may say so, this is a strength rather than a weakness. Your thoughts emerge from the pages as I imagine they occurred to you. Your writing is therefore fresh and spontaneous - whilst retaining an overall structure by its chapters.

For me, the effect is of a personal contact. It is almost as if I am reading a long letter from a friend. I'm certain that I am not alone in this experience. Whilst the style is, of course, particularly engaging, I hope it will have the consequence of assisting your readers, (as it has certainly helped me) both to a greater understanding of Asperger's syndrome and to a determination to approach those who may experience it in way which is appropriate to their wishes and, most importantly, to recognise that none of us are 'defined' by our 'condition' - whatever that may be.

Thank you once again.

Kevin.

Foreword.

I am returning to College soon 'Guildford College' Surrey - so into better my 'Maths & English'. Pre - GCSE / GCSE... part-time.

My use throughout this my 2nd Book you are about to Read, isn't perfect regarding Grammar - Punctuation - Spelling; preference to use English rather than American English, isn't always case.

Punctuation I am aware of, quotation marks - speech marks - brackets - bold black highlights - No use of Indents - Paragraphs of my own design; and much more I am sure irritants; that a well versed man shall pick up unto. The spoken meaning of my Autistic Punctuation is in my language. As is my Grammar and use of Vocabulary.

This does all require I fall in line universally across the board of said Standard English; and so it is one day It is my hope, I may re-edition my first example, when better knowledge is my revised friend.

The shear scale of my books size, has meant attention too details isn't a 'time factor I'm blessed with', the headache involved, with so much of an outer world pushing me away; from what I love to do.

My personal choice Autistic uses Capital letters in Words randomly, and have cut down their use in free flow - where possible.

I hope this all shall not spoil, your own enjoyment.

Chapter 1.

Sun's Poem

My Autistic Cliché: I am In this World, I am not of it.

The Sun sitting up so high, I want to look up, keep my energy's high.

The Reality is the Sun's colour is not a colour my eyes tell me it is, all that is really there, Science & Nature, things that don't care, simply no fizz.

The Spirit without me 'sees the Sun' not in a physical body matter, such as I do. And no Spirit at all sees nothing, no matter, red herring, calamity, a man with no face, tracing paper that won't trace.

The Tilt I see the Sun from, is a position it stays, I leave it turned on.

A normal person without God by his side, sees not one position of our Sun, his a logical thinker, he said please, throw away fun.

For everyday - for the rest of his life, the Sun kept changing formation, he would not see it as I do, it's why he's unsettled - he's got them changing blues.

One Sun settled. Unchanged. Your Asperger's love. He wakes up, feels happy cause nothing's changed, non altered love he felt yesterday - still remains. Today, tomorrow the day after, limit is bird free the sky.

There's no need to do more than required, already he's there. I shake my Umbrella, the Weather Flood Rains blow her inside out, this is God's fury, humanity's stink.

The poems I wrote left best, made real man's, pleasing blue ink.

It is easy, it is simple, it's what rings fabric with me, but oh no more this World wants you climbing their trees - so you just follow thy they.

Gone are the days of quiet library's Sherlock Holmes, bread and dripping, inter-war years, further back - reading by tallow candle lights, authority figures developing a turn around fear.

Then. Popular Dance music destroyed it, dead, like the Dodo, extinct the traditional man became.

'When, where,' one phase ends. We're told - a new one starts.

Hello and welcome to my Second Book. (*The 2nd Encounter - Volume 2*).

I am Simon R. Newell.

My poems made from dancing nonsense. A.S. awkwardness.

My poems were standardized good - and so like a good standard. Antique young, my collection had no value relative. Fore they were all but 1 week old.

Though passable reading with one eye squinted, made the Mona Lisa sing. 'They had no strength, no age,' she said of my Poems - merely one week old.

Welcome. I am Simon - please come inside. Lock thy door - this is my World a step further on. Wipe feet thine, Shalom thou resides present in book 2's corridors - ((No more Secrets)) Series.

Many a persons' gained enjoyment from my master piece poems, my one week old poems gained momentum, now they peaked. One month old.

These poems gained strength - curiously cause they did not move - like watching a scary film, back rigid - rigor mortis.

Imagine the activity all around the World, what has happened what has not. The things we broke - to kept solid rock.

The dying/rebirth of new babies. The different time zones we are split up under - Caucasian races - Asian, White, African, Mixed race, Pakistan, Hispanic, Latin lineage, Indian, so on.

This World - 'had got busy'. While sleeping states in the quiet rooms.

Surrounded my poems in free love, my ignorance child spirit protected - away from bustling outside World.

2 Months past - my poems did not move remained sat - same spot.

The Wars went on through the Eras of time, people married, fell in love, hurricanes, bad weathers, monuments - greened flaked.

Dreams destroyed - heavy monumental statues standing crumbled, the ones you walked past every day. Echoed out. Forever.

Divorce's separated, now single.

People you knew once alive in your lifetime. 'We held think were strong,' like noble men of our time, now deceased (too early), close friends, family, associates. Lord Admiral Nelson, Queen Victoria. No longer making - forever.

Though hard people, perhaps simply strong people. Non-famous, (close people too you - 'they were') and all you knew divided famous, Infamous.

Wanted you did - no end, just friends. Outside body grown old remains growth young - the same young you was always.

History 'read' documented - 'about you' - was not just seen only as (Grey reading) we'd hope. A family member you was, among them in those days. Porthole periods in history highlighted - those crowds these days... you'd be laughing at such antiquity's, suggestions placed

Importances - from the shadows.

Historians grow in - sought after knowledge. Needs not a heavy thumb - in all we do.

Declaring this is how it played out - exactly printed.

Upon gathered, relied on information's intelligence. Yet no script accurate enough we can deduce as played out in (each individual - persons of history), singular through. What he tells you - (just what went on - happened).

Became a Shadow of themselves (they had - they were), though as much as we cared about, those we call 'them', these figures of brass, they still had the ruling thumb - over their people, as weak as thee stood.

The solid strong political figures, swapping roles, becoming the poor down-trodden people - reaching out gaining support - divides them.

Us we became rich. In heart, I said I will not change.

The prim and ever so proper - Archery, the croquet, the Polo games on horse back, a day at the Stables dear fellow, the jolly good shows, the ever so dandy, noses in the air, her name's Candy - you know the ones, the ever so rich.

We are a family unit in it together to the divided end - not matter your status, (say come again). A jolly holiday with Mary - Dick van dyke. So no wonder that it's Mary that we love.

The likes of the bad starters in life (the unlucky), not so fortunate, clubbed battered tree-like hands. Made me cry 'love they had', they wanted for nothing.

They're homeless - the broken - the morning hurting. Didn't care to be the best-est Musicians - information theory's, was more than he could bear in care.

He already was - stricken with worry the way this World puts 'an emphasis on his heart', not needing to lose any more of his own hair.

My Poems were now 3 months old, my mind had grown - older, slow, candid.

I - In-sighted re-read, my poems through. It was not like before, it was like these poems - (were new) fresh - not read - not all with Rhythm constituted throughout, embedded full double bed-spread.

I could not remember (values) I placed - I'd not read them in a while. My poems did not devalue Interest, what I absorbed again today, I know when happy with my work spouts clear, goose bumps, hair static, chill in the air.

Butterfly cramps somersaulted - a held joy in my stomach, energy working like the end of the River - has somewhere to go.

(Turns - you saved - before going ahead), gives your early bird worm efforts you put in. (You creased in) - early kink by physical kink worked.

No wonder your River shouts like this life has no end. A beginning, a middle is all (here and now) - the (end), also a (continuation presence) a moving beginning - folded in rivers, washed rapid, wash quiet.

Another day ends, 'the future unreachable', always it's effort right now.

The River effort is your future - no other rivers taking you. Direct futures reached only via here and now effort affects.

When you make arrival to your future, other futures are running into other futures, awkward. Rivers running into each other - never knowing which way's out.

Following your nose like a good Marine - hears, smells, talks his way out of trouble. Flotation devices just will not do alone.

This marine did not workout - in with other marines, for nothing no how to say ((this mission ends)) - he's one of the men, charity Volunteering - watch out river's bend.

Comrades do all of this for you. This was all going on

when my poems, 'I locked in a suitcase', had turned 4 months old.

The strengths Prevailing and failing - was History gone on.

My Poems - my wheel spokes awkward - (survived). What with screaming children too loud, running around homes, far too proud.

Bad language people getting angry - families in turmoil.

The flickering street light which flicked a beam of light through your curtains at night - (nobody fixed), was again (history changed) new formulated words, new conversations now taking place. Your otherwise divulged concentrations affected - taking away focus - you wouldn't have otherwise lost.

Places - your movements - your language - all altered. 'Your future' - by one ever so Innocent flickering street lamp.

Had everything been as it should - ((new bulb, no flicker)), your future untold undisturbed. Future futures, rolling new time lines - larger than a (Graham's number) - is you in - left Natural.

The Council would not spread money, some things happen this way, history walking the diverted paths.

Neglected, cause no one ((can afford to pay)). The good and bad emerging in broken - and all mended paths, (helps on one side. Hinders on one side), (middle lines - copping) - a collection of unknown help and hinders - future story's shared.

The Car that shone a beam of light through your bedroom's window, hit one wall climbing high. Descending shadow patterns were cast, like a protractor in your pencil case - radiating radius the ceiling's sky, your safe snug night comforts, security warmth of family ties.

On a school's wooden desks - tell me how many children have sat here - counting the array of bubblegum that's stuck to an underside gloom - gone so hard - you'd think it was: P 38/P 40 (Car filler).

A car crept in your ((Close - at night)), you know you're half awake half dreaming, deep in thought, sudden jerks of movement make you jump.

Like radiators cooling down where she got so hot, the thoughts you were lost in, now matter no not. The old wooden floorboards creak more at night - breaking you. Your heart skips one last time.

Noticeably so quiet - all noises distancing away in thin air - drunk men - couples ranting a split.

The (room's dark) - you are dead still in your bed.

The car outside is reflecting you light across your patterned ceiling - creeping on gentle best behaviour he crawls - a timid man, career minded - suit hanging back seat window, specially designed hook.

Waking his neighbour's fleet - not beat - feet - foot easy on clutch.

Not everyone works funny hours, so not everyone appreciates. Still lying in your bed the intriguing noise, a loud speaker made amplified upon the rest of the 'Close' sleeping.

(Times) - your night experiences - laying spread-eagle in bed or silencing you - Cars crawling engine - by 10 - double this figure.

You hit closer understandings how now - Asperger sufferers in the day time, try keeping their engine noise low - the way he/I will quiver. Only finds our efforts in vain lost hugely. Usually from an over-aggressive loud persuasion we are said too. ((Just follow along with)).

Yet strangely these persons loud disturbing - in day time periods - insist on quiet neighbours come Night.

> A.S. Autism insists Night and Day concludes - 'quiet pictures'.

Asked we mix in - mingle. Sounds a good idea you might think right. (Yet makes matters worse) since they, the Normal N.T.s discover we reside - not of their makings.

And so we A.S. are easily dismantled for not showing a shared fitting In. Not on purpose we do it. We simply have a motor cortex wired free of togetherness, ((others want)).

This car shadowing me, lights my ceiling's Rosetta and distributed 4 corners - who had a late night board meeting one assumed, stayed an extra hour round his Girlfriend's perhaps, the funny hours he worked - he was sure he'd wangle it creeping home.

2 minutes drilling a quiet stance took 20, making dead sure - his driver's side don't slam.

One car - one door handle. 2 minutes ultra slow motion of handle movement so as not to disturb - ((plus checks - clocks him time)) - quieter than a classical piece by George. F. (Handel).

My Poems reach 5 Months and 4 days old.

Asperger Awkwardness evidently left in all nooks and crannies - spotted by them in the high seats, pure in-sighted awkwardness he and I spectrum trained, vowed vouched no removal - until Asperger conditions cared - care is given. A place where Asperger suffering reduces to a resembling Normal to N.T.s. or our Normal.

A.S. Persons' - he sees it as - he's planted his trees, with asked for (more powers given), snips and prunes - too his own. Awkward delight, climates he favours.

Much has happened (pressed on time) - from the life birth, my poems were born. Some I hammered out, sometimes I was torn.

I wrestled with gravity, time and again, I sank low key moments - (blocked thoughts), struggling I sure as H*ll never did - ((gave In)).

Waiting on something more, instinctive I knew. I was there - the vision Asperger's is me, or it is not - I easily tear.

I am the creator master chauvinist barbaric pig, you grow impatient despair - my Asperger Ways.

Casting your Fisher's Rod out - one last time. One last time. And no one last time again. Building up a pendulum swing in you - so eyes forward, swing thrust cast. Zip sound sore finger - watch your cast sing.

4 ounce weight shall do nicely Sir - I see it still moving... I think this one will go far.

My Poems lost my Interest nothing more would I do, no ratchet handle strength of mind is pulling them through.

Best walk away, life is not my revolving door - on my terms. Travelling light through only one spectrum means - why A.S.? (Stay insistent). Your Asperger clue.

Well I tried Acoustic guitaring - wrote books - gone fishing. Had writer's block. Walked away, experience enter clean feathers.

Am I writing to you non confident. Then confidence showing through - again Asperger's is your clue.

My Poems are 2yrs, 1 week - plus I don't know - 42 days old.

You know the maths, (it's an Asperger's thing), hidden clues.

My Poems swam older and older swamps, I had done become a lot in my life. Sacked from jobs, had girlfriends turn the other cheek/blind eyes.

I am with you in birth my Asperger cousin softly said.

Then you get Those saying - they're here for you, ((if and when - you want me)) such like - N.T. Normal types.

((You know where I am - where I'll be - types)) that don't give credentials handed - honesty's thread.

So A.S. designed as I am - (coupled to my girlfriend) - any given girlfriend - quote as: Normal girlfriend material - boyfriend. As the case may bid.

Has me saying:

OK look ((I want you)). You get this - fashioned with sincerity I slung an honesty bridge open.

I ask you, (as, I the man) opened the (first door). Did they/did you - climb In, extend me an excitement level on par the same or close - I radiated?

The same ones saying they're here for me - quote: 'if and when - I want them'.

I have to say sorry. Not from my A.S. perspective no.

I found more honesty I gave, in a World dishonest only strengthened my resolve - (I am A.S kind) - built this way.

You're a (Woman in a Moment) I said. So she said yes. So please Simon - can we leave it right there?

This was a relief my ears picked up unto Hear.

Thank God pleased. Asperger sensitivity wobbly; no more scares.

We are boys, men - the only moving dominantly correct same. (Asperger Normals) - share common recognition.

Asperger orientated though stubborn - are Fair - Fair - Fair drummed In.

The Poems set out in the books are mine. Was Thunder and Lightning fun my heart this time around lived, a side too of me (unsynced) - measured with added not precise - unplanned Rhythms.

Synced Rhythms Poetry - comes cleaner crisper sure. However, I like a choice running my gauntlet free rhythm exposed - bang on the drum - strong weak tangled parallels.

I was this always forever: (an only person who knew - of open rhythmic broken existence). A.S can be both Rhythmic strong - Rhythmic paths broken - yet seldom do we become only one with conviction, unless it is a (compulsion, an Interest). We are supported with backings up to the hilt - care reaching circulating Interest my fingers burdened - a non performance asked - I give - only then.

Like a girl lost in the Woods, she was not SAS trained.

Smoke signals, showing the messages in her mind, in my Poem - breaks Rhythm the trials; reality brought.

God said Simon let it blossom, let it go, you do not have a singular care in the World my child, nor worry finishing, finished. As 'placed emphasis' on the glass tidy.

The disgusted displeased people running parallel curriculums to 'unequal approvals'. Congratulate your high praise of never quite fixated forever in one truth within.

The mind requires your faithful mind loyal, (one picked side (family - team - party), and now your not change loyalties - to go higher in your own personal experience, chosen already people you represents.

You shall lose and win without the destruction of your new experimental courses - changing your loyalties. You fight for your side through thick and thin.

You accept defeat as much as you do accept gains. Wins you claim. Neither reduce your fight the person you are. This is how you think.

Don't laugh or snigger at others' defeats - to boost your own party - family - teams' morale. We're in this together we hadn't forgot.

Relaxed path brings 2 elements: unlevelled/levelled randomly free to go higher. Stop the challenges - (bring on the Accepts).

The Key is -(love unlevelled awkward persona's), before placing the clean palatables; as A.S.s better way to go.

Given this choice you are more inclined to learn both languages, rather than! one seen as the force dominant to be reckoned with.

Lose the Character you thought I was in Book 1. The Plain Truth. Mostly that was just low sketching Foundations, bring you through, (there I stayed). Out Rhymed - out of common Rhythm. Awkward Tension - broke tension. Rhymed, lost Rhyme.

Low functioning is, I declare - my rest easy home. A place unhinged no burden pressure performance, not required.

I find enjoyment living silly - (Low Functioning). I am happy there.

I find enjoyment (High Functioning). I am happy there. I am not a man born for one or the other as preference-d. I am a feeder born of 2 Worlds. I cannot be (only one). I need both kidneys.

I can not expand my High Functioning self if indeed you rejected me as Low Functioning. I care to be both. I cannot expand my progression unless you're giving me your conviction - beloved. Low Functioning equal.

New minority brave ways sliding through, here on the other side. This is job stay.

I can take you so far In - hard efforts shining through me, shining through you. I am not back stepping to be more than I am, so moving slow home in ((Low Function)) - is progress not seen ridiculed we'd hope, by powers who keep us, grasping foundations of us - they dashed hadst kept zipped - we let the Winners through (so I walked home to lose), reasons of healing reasons of strength.

Arrogance is fine, it has carried you this far. Arrogance in the good sense, harmless sense. Splash/hoover, cleaning my Car.

It is nice when I see you're the Teacher. It is not all one sided, left purposely loose soil.

My own Tractor covers vast farm patches, 'missing out' all corners covered Story. (Over time) I am not granted guarantee. I effort A.S only.

Just don't lose sight of the planter's simple ways. He got you thinking, made you who you are; turnouts today.

My Poems over time - now 10 years old lost lots of dust, bent corners, cat's hair, ear wax, man's lipstick, triangle corners, temporary book markers.

These poems have seen a lot, heard a lot. People leaving and entering rooms, conversations gone on.

Quietly built in strength my poems served one purpose; surviving strong in a 10th year.

Time surrounding us this Moment, no matter our different ages - we remain together like glue.

This day we are together unchanged. (All days).

Different ages stages. I am/you - is age the same - (today's age).

We are Family Aspergic/non Aspergic.

One day it reached the year (2032); man has successfully orbited a trajectory to Mars on numerous occasions.

We divide our Inhabitants upon 2 Worlds.

Steven Hawking's set - ((2 Wormholes in place)) - our saved manned fuel.

And my Poems took the brunt of the Force, set backs - knocks - good fortunes.

I played Guitar before I wrote Books, master Musician 'given control - I use free' my mind's expenses.

A newly crafted World - wants to etch away at you - till you fit glove replica mould of the people you despise.

Rather than protesting my fight a guitar education in me - soaring sour, deteriorating indecisive support - (I built 10 years strong - under Labour).

Meant instead I lost valuable time, stuck in a rut doing nothing, progressing my education forward Acoustic guitar, (stopped suddenly) no backing, no support, problems - that to continue denoted I was lazy. A mind framework I am wired under, contributes effort compassed on (freewill learning). Giving back in society's hub 'the many ways', prosperity, good work, produces a democratic people with options. Reaching same results, better results from - seen working practical products, wise options handed by the high councils - money not the denominator to your success ((just left options)) - democratic people choose free will.

Contribution of economics economy - is **one way** methodology; not granted a human reliance.

Unfortunately money dictates your willingness; to give back - your society within fruit bearing ripe. Fruits from natural you.

Deep bore, wild boar options, gave healthy strengths (contributed to us), the ordinary folk - my World turning around (**effort**) - not centred on money as mandatory themes.

It costs money to produce money which in turn costs (wasted effort), (technology - advancements in Sciences - Engineering - as two examples) suffers by the laid energy - man power. (Now not there) not now benefiting man's progressed doors.

Understanding (**Materials**) our planet. Materials **you Craft** - paid for, distributed by (Mother's Earth) not Mother's man - just so as long as you **pay effort** - do **justice to.** (Mother Earth's - Materials).

Is payment due enough - '**is paid.**'

A heart is shaped so you don't alter. And since money is not the natural heart shape - it is no wonder (**Work** produced **turned out**) in this World - is not Natural Sawdust - it's extra taken time (wasted). Time calculated - ((**effort/ time** - diverted wasted forever - logging ((what you owe)) - counting your stack of Coins - money eats away at '**time.**'

Whereas (direct **effort** gives) quicker efficient paid contribution back - to a Work hard Society working together.

Counting - **good effort owed** - as a freer way to pay - is both less pressured - less time consuming labelling items for Sale. Less Logging accounts upon account books piling high. Less data entry on Computers filing spreadsheets.

In short less checks in a monetary world means! (more efforts we give) as a people.

And so 'Time' - handed back.

Options is where it's at. Democratic relations with your kind of people.

My Guitar Life was thrown away dedication 12hr 16hr days educating myself. Most days for **10 years education** thriving crystal clear - theoretical and practical usages, now lost.

The drive required - the momentum required keeping up 'high Guitar Educations' indoctrinated In.

(Gone) under new governance.

Money was now regarded the higher priority in governed powers 2010 on wards - over priorities money I had, already Invested (in Self Education). Asked to walk away from all I spent Investing bettering myself. Asked to walk away from already embedded Educations built of me instilled.

A job (Full time) - they want for me paying Tax contributions (not making the best of me) a derailment of what '**they** see as **right**', and in some, not all ways it is! has me paying in (a - rerouted) mindset.

Full time work wastes paperwork; people not getting on with me.

Materials related to Guitar - **Books - DVDs - CDs.** I built up over time - benefits no one taking me away from my tools, my materials, my diet - I asked once in Ernest I be allocated space, time around me. Asperger necessities.

Expansion environments Information. Learning minds take on board - (I use); equates to this laid Table undisturbed.

Produced - **Guitar Educational packages**, made. Wastes their time/my time. In, (Products they sold me).

Given me no benefit - (left) hanging around expensive

materials - laid helpless in my room.

How I think a man with my Syndrome; has 'this affect'.

Some agree, some decline to pass powers... some dislodge your 'paid for path', some hesitated - some dominated - some mounted the high horses.

Some want to dis-spell you of any preconceived Ideas. I cannot switch lanes change automatic.

Guitar songs broken in maples rosemary neck - is rich, free contribution.

All songs mine smashed guitars. Durdle door rocks.

Weymouth's West coast - (songs play) ghost like now forward.

I am like you now, forward. A big builder's fluorescent jacket - the smell of a Worker's Union, steel toe-capped boots.

A Slave back in gone Cotton pickin' Blues days 1910s, singing my Chant workers song character.

My Builder's Jacket, it smelt of angry faces. In this together.

Awkward poetry ends.

Chapter 2.

Keeping the rhyme. 3rd poem

Guitar. Job-focused-Interviews. Lord Mayors.

Simon Guitar Teacher.

B.B King loves to play the Blues, he loves our 'Lucille' for she is guitar broken through songs through, this guitar's wood, got history blues ma'am great use of vibrato, bends, trills. Mrs Brown.

One day I reached ages of 44 to 65 - I was now a working man, working for benefits.

Distributed leaflets for my own 'benefits', such as we do.

5 years ago I made a pact with our Job Centre. They were real nice, to the relaxed powers letting me know ever so.

Working Asperger clues - (with me).

Really working my prospective job-lot movements, knowing I could break, I could crumble. Lisa my Job Focused Interviewer called my ticket and sat me down.

We had coffee & scones brought in just for occasion, she even said Simon, loosen your Shoe laces. They were a bit tight.

So this I agreed.

She said Simon what do you know, what can we agree.

So I took a deep breath, built tension, before release spoke my words.

Lisa Swang swung her bottom lip - left right hips, swivel chair, disturbances fixate me on.

Thanks a bunch Lisa inviting me to your office today.

She didn't seem Religious - from her left hip swing.

Then a glint in my eye meeting hers - shined safely a St Christopher; she shone.

Criss-crossing her legs once every 4 seconds - pivoting her hips - I'd got a glimmer of her St Christopher, one last time.

My eyes were going all over the show, Lisa pivoting her ground.

I said, Lisa. I met The Lord Mayor, 17th Feb 14.

Through a friend of my sister Hayley named Nassar. Liberal democrat, same as what the Lord Mayor of Portsmouth practice's In.

I am Labour myself, not sure I'm even - (that).

Labour / Green / Ukip / S.n.p something like this.

I said Lisa, listen - you know the last time we met, way back - October the 4th 2013, my memory serving me correct.

You said what you doing then Simon, to look for work - job focused Interview, (focused alright), watching her swing left to right.

Damn focus I was getting, but hey this is serious stuff, so let's do as the title tells us: Focus - no fuss.

So I said - Lisa, you said to me, Simon what you doing to look for work - (then).

And last time we met I said to you, Lisa - I was considering a conversation we discussed.

About me being - (Simon / Teacher). I shall work for my benefits - in a School, that is close to where I live, wherever this maybe.

And you will have a **Word** with the (Governor's board) of the School; in seeing if they require a Supplied Teacher at this time. Namely me.

I was a bit nervous about Teaching, yet also with drive I am good for the expansion.

Music don't have Rhythm, set out on - 'blackboards' broken white chalk.

And why I mentioned to you, teaching Junior School kids, not full grown adult panda's. It requires confidence building. I require a start somewhere elbow room.

Today at my - Work. F. Interview, on 24th February 2014, it is fair to say - Lisa! 'it's been a long while since our last contact'.

You said you'd get back to me within 2 to 3 weeks about a job in a School - as 'Simon Guitar Teacher' or Mr Newell - ((we meet - see my pupils)), here take a seat.

Lisa you're - (nicest Interview lady ever met), and here's a copy of my 1st book signed by Author, Simon R Newell.

Listen - had a re-think Lisa, although (my idea) I brought forward to you, placed in your lap, about the Teacher business, previously talked through ideas grew.

Actually 2nd thoughts way my nerves blew; a Classroom full of kids, keeping their focused attention, impressing the Guitar is hard to do.

Forgiven you are - I am of the Era - 'of', Thing one & Thing 2. (Cat in the Hat).

I am a free Spirit Teaching man/boy, with a pie-graph chart. Guitar Theory's too scary, on young minds.

And should I show weakness, (in a love song I sing) played on guitar. The hard cruel world, cannot accept (love in songs), such as I do.

Schools have a Regimented hardness, that my music is not about, need I say more! Asperger's your clue.

I racked my brains for you Lisa, got real excited with you today. Looking at you squarely in ones eyes, I say -

say yeah, oh yes Lisa, that's the (Job for me).

Actually - believing it so.

The Thrill of my 45 minute job focused Interview ends. I walk back home, buying can of coke/cheap energy drink.

My Asperger's starts playing up. I realize how perfect I would need Shape up. Fulfilling my Acoustic dreams - job.

Yes. Music can be taught, especially by a Teacher born into Music, I wasn't born this luxury, brought up In Music.

Advising any young kids, whether you come from a (Musical Family) or (Non Music Families), should music ring your passion, and you want too be a Teacher, then realize your dreams, quicker smart.

Live and breathe Music. Music in your bed clothes at night - set the alarm for an early rise 0700hrs.

Train on Guitar at least 12 hours a day - this is the dedication we talk about. I started learning Guitar at the ages of 29/30 roughly, back.

We didn't have Welfare issues with Governing bodies', that's when - I was training myself 12hrs a day. Religiously, strictly. I once was real good.

Though the Level of my greatness changed through the years, depending on what life's throwing at us today.

Concentration is what you will need in your Guitar's kit bag, if you are wanting to make progress here, and I do.

Unhealthy eating drugs through the years has had its toll on my body, along with cruel World at times.

So in light with consideration, I thought why not just teach infant/junior kids. Although my knowledge of Guitar might bamboozle a young mind, not an intention. I am just A.S. so let it weigh heavy.

Had I had clear intentions of becoming the highly polished Guitar Teacher required of you today, I'd relay to you - (really not what I am about).

I am too free in head, 41 years old.

The battles are best served with your New young minded Teacher, you can draft in for such threads, so this leads me too say, old or young, all experience - leads through this - ((**door**)).

So with this in mind Lisa, I have decided to be - what the World wants of me, a Leaflet distributor, for the Liberal democrats Volunteer, to earn my benefits, rest of my 20 or so years please.

Then I can retire - when an old boy, and play guitar how I wanted too when I 1st set out.

So Lisa, leaflet distributor - can you swing it.

The Lord Mayor and I spoke as you know, she was very helpful, toad in the hole.

She is setting up a Volunteer's Job for me as a distributor of Leaflets.

I gave Lisa my sister's (friend's number) - Nassar.

Can Job-centre please 'liaise with' governing bodies of the Lord Mayor. Say yes, Simon is happy too take this agreed role?

I heard nothing back :-(

More awkward rhymes. 3rd Poem continued.

My Guitar life took such a battering, all my hard work. I studied hard - slaved, nights, days, weeks years, decades on, was to become a crushed car, no more sensitivity applied than at a Rubbish car tip.

So best it was - I close the door on something I never wanted give up.

The Pipers whistle has blown in a World unfair, nice people caring - people I gave it up for.

Your turn too fill my boots up, you be the Musician awhile, it is little more than a hobby just about now.

Hurts abandoning my post - to let go, less hours granted gives only (lesser Musicianship).

My music wasn't wasted, gave many a person's enjoyment through the years.

From built used carpentry skills, Guitar projects I turned around. I made Guitar easy to learn.

To date although neglected I have written 14 Songs handwritten using (Guitar Keys) in varying ways.

Wrote my own (Chord Progressions), thrown in a little melody - man oh man leaves me hungry more even at my age 41 to 44.

Again, No Backing support followed me provided, so downed tools, downed (strings) regrettably.

Enough's enough. I'm no quitter Characteristic notable in this Syndrome A.S. you know.

So with the way things panned out, 'reverts' unintelligent Simon again.

People seem to like/love you, when you don't show intelligence. Is this love? No it is not.

Is it love, as persons' who pose - to be your friends, love you (only when) - you're unintelligent? I personally don't believe so.

Is it love when people who pose to be with you, love you equally as much - (Intelligent or unintelligent)? Yes. In this case - Love true - Is.

So I'm still sat down the damn Job Centre with Lisa. I ask her, listen up - I pose a proposition, left suggest in your lap.

Yes she says: Go ahead Simon. **Thank you Lisa.**

What's troubling you Simon?

Well I have decided I don't want to work for money. I don't want to be your plain ordinary (Clock in), run of the mill person rough litter, who is happy to follow the crowds.

I wish (he) - referenced as the (World) - loosely spoke

- joined us all on freedoms trail - circulations clean heart.

Stating his Job-centre want-ages unharnessed - no boundaries - added control entrust, a juggler of his own Time-sheets.

So please listen carefully, I only can say this once, cause to repeat myself, is hurting my energy's core.

Yes Simon... !

Lisa look, I want too earn my benefits via Voluntary measures the last half my life.

A job delivering leaflets for our Liberal Democrat friends, Labour/Greens call it what will, to making Bird Boxes - free minded ideas, suits me down the Ground.

I don't have to work a 40 hour week - since I enlist other jobs - totalling hours, worked in.

A Solution Job-centre - (agreed), haunting Interviews cease, process benefit both us all.

Delivering leaflets, squeaking gates, angry dog houses. A far field; Surrey Hampshire areas.

Time scales I work each week month and year, shall differ each week, never quite the same ever. Interests juggled - keeper maintaining levels mine high.

Mobile phone handy sat in Rucksack of mine, whilst out on deliveries, (should you juggle exciting ideas new), changes re-routed, uprooted, making foreplay a 'freshman' energized. Sings less focused Interviews.

So One Job possible Simon, Volunteer Leaflet distributor services you offer, Liberal Democrats nice yellow orange colours sewn in jacket and Shirt.

Like motorcycles group. Simon's Patch.

Though to be fair, I heard nothing back from our Lord Mayor of Portsmouth busy booked annual schedules perhaps, one assumes.

Delivering for Labour/Greens possibly. I'd love to deliver for our Mr J. Corbyn.

Maybe leaflets to distribute is 'not for me' after all.

What else can I do to look in your eyes, standing tall.

I tried Self educating guitar, making (Guitar Aids) help others, (to stay this best), and you said this is something we cannot allow you do.

A (Secondary Job) Volunteering in Nature - 3rd, fourth or fifth, sets free Simon. Additional jobs supplementing your one main hub centred theme, (under a mind) - fighting in Asperger Survival.

You are willing in your agenda, active awkward prepared, you enjoy work 40 hour lengths a week should your body allow !

Pleasing those (worked in your opposite) - you do.

Boxed in working frames of 40 hours only 'does not' work how you grow, especially when your help you give freely, is a make-shift of 20 hour, 40 hour 60 hour, 80 hour weeks - free patterns with easier unknown in-between hours. You set deadlines the body yours talks. Simon.

Working harder in Voluntary you do Simon, than any tax complication world, show more productiveness assertiveness, as opposed snared heavy one way work loaded jobs.

Flourish your better thoughts, creates your better works, Voluntary free movement (yet again) however Simon, sorry! something we cannot allow you do for reasons mapped.

Do you have something else you'd like to do Simon?

Yes Lisa. You know all problems I gave to why in why - 'why it was' - a bad idea to become (Simon Guitar Teacher)?

Yes Simon!

Well I'd like to become a Guitar Teacher in another

formation, what with pressure ladled on me, stresses my inner mechanical mind signals tangled, exacerbating a person I cannot be for you accelerates my failings. Heart palpitations panic attacks unless obeying our mind instructive we find no harmony. (None).

A.S people cannot stray from a (Conditioned) - head- mind- body- legs- feet- arms- hands- fingers- coordination, built diagnosis, describing their default position. And when we do guess what, we crumble.

An outcome working against my asked for conditions results: 'Meltdowns' - Depression - lost Interest, dysfunctioning our first language - and we say no this is not on then we are looked at oddly for showing fury.

Suggestive too you - you let me grow in life, showing thee what I am capable of do in World, not - what not, you calling all the shots.

Well how you going to implement this carried out Simon?

Good Question Lisa.

Here is additional voluntary job adage extra jobs tangled together barbs wire thoughts entwined, bird's nest messy making up in mind totals, jobs ticked possible.

I forever have shown you - my hard work, 'my hand' now what must I do? (here is my proposal).

Look my head is wise council Encyclopedia wealth. Information's yes? Guitar Theory one examples.

So what better way than to allowance me pour out my head format Writer A.S Syndrome Guitar Books - for the rather Stranger of thinkers - those like me.

Each Book I master shall take 1 year 5 months a quickest deadline. Influx focus plotting a damn good sketched outline, advanced beforehand and in the mean time plotting pinpointed accurate diagrams continuous - the very obscure shall find easy.

This shall stimulate with degree - help people never Struggle again.

You say: Simon, you earn your benefits by helping others - written Books. Not just Guitar Books, A.S. Syndrome Books, inclusive.

I have nothing to benefit myself letting you down - so (I wont let you down).

I've shown you handful few pins head of intelligence, shaped no other way fashioned no other way.

Said gentle: you can cut this pie 2 ways.

Yes Simon, I am setting wheels in motion as we speakeasy ... or no Simon - keep thinking baby, re-think.

Chapter 3.

The Spectrum come. Medical Professional.

Asperger's - including the Autistic Spectrum, '**is best described**' (**by** Doctors/Professionals akin), who eat sleep live with the Spectrum.

They see more Asperger's persons (in their day) than I meet within months, they can really give you the professional slang's used in the Medical fields, better than we Asperger can - tongued loosely.

A Doctor, come Professional, come Specialist, shall have does have more leverage, ((a longer crowbar)), fortified in Theory & medical journals practises studies observed.

One Doctor takes in studying of the Asperger subject, reports back too his colleagues. The comparison of notes begins, this is similar too how a (Musician) eats, sleeps, breathes Music.

Our (Doctor friends) - experts in the field become taught first base Foundations principled by say the: Colleges. Further Higher Educations. Universities. Special board of members, what have you.

Then he's set free from 'nestling of College Lecturers' teaching him - who were taught say 10yrs previous with (provided studies **updated**) - upon curriculum necessitates kept in line advances.

Mix and mingled in (formulations) stooped. (Principles and Symptoms recognized) - by governing bodies and members concerned. Examples you look for perhaps. Detailed analysis, experience in studies, '**they do know about**'.

You see quickly how complicated it can get through

specific (highways and byways) of the College - Uni thinker, (all it Relates).

Asperger individuals and the Medical profession (are a **secret team**), 'not connected' to the same train of thought.

We as Asperger Autistics - (need the Professional teams), as much as the Professional teams need us.

Asperger persons' and Medical Doctors in varying fields catering (are **not** colleagues - this we know), they're not Enemies either, they are **associates** to the Spectrum.

The Asperger's (job) as a representative to his fellow cousin Asperger 'helps the Doctors' (keep it simple). Reasons en-route why books written by Asperger people themselves (diagnosed), give over simple, (hands on) approach - answers.

This is why seemingly there are Doctors (and not just Doctors) - '**recognition's** - in ordinary folk', best **highlighted** to giving the ((**Informative approach**)).

Furthering your knowledge finding a (**Course**) topical Interest (**for you**) in say ((**Spectrum disorders**)) Asperger's / Autism at an Institution establishment near you or further afield! Helps Common found structures build knowledge.

Yet through my harmonious reaction I find nothing In common boxed with another Autistic; as I am sure many N.T.s shall not be studied same matching simply because it is proven they are labelled Normals. All this might suggest a lean towards different Characters we are placed; not so much the traffic lights we Spectrum a function said too Share; with untold Symptoms building the Model human we perspire a wanted difference Individual.

Just one 'pick-up Information taken' adds and subtracts shapes we display matches on thrust hurling towards the 'Models' we build as reliable equations too solve Answers Answered rolled within no matter your colouring Spectrum Identification; is too me at least unquestionable Art Work. And therefore logical wasn't looking to be discovered.

There is not One Answer expressing as One Artist - One Picture Complete. Only one Artist expressed as a Picture left too dazzle many unravelled thoughts illogical with no wanted Answers; so much so he dropped his own Keys down the drain; and why perhaps when looking for the wholesome Answers we all Identify as there simply isn't none to be found; Autistic man/ Normal man muddled on many decrees.

No one gives you better lived-in experience than the man who knows 'with A.S.' Like an Electric Guitar (Fender Stratocaster), a player with good (Chops) knows. So does A.S.

You see, an Aspergic's Electric Guitar is extra worn In, than the expensive guitar a Doctor can afford.

Oh yes, a Doctor can play (sure I know), though his Guitar isn't worn in enough to be a Soldier of Asperger dug in deep. Foxhole. Enemy flank 500yrds, entering the North West Territory.

Although! where Doctor Medical teams climb in, get on board with their family Asperger (is - they live out within situations occupying 'Asperger presence days' in their today).

They observe huge numbers - with selected added Specialized cases. Asperger people assessed under patterns them - (day by day) taking very detailed notes off their own back before comparing (notes) recorded awareness, their team clans share.

'Answers Research achieved, is on honest watches' seeing lived in A.S.s diagnosed - through one observer only. (One Doctor) qualified clues tell tell signs. This same doctor breaks away from the pack researching in a humanistic quality.

All Nurses and Doctors (have fun learning), same as Asperger do.

(This is **similarity** we do share), yet are we the same? ((nope)).

Every weekday **nights**, (**meetings** were called) from (Hotel

Autistic Hospital - 10pm till 12:30am).

All briefcases carried became thrown in the meetings centre room, left of middle side - in room **stacked.**

A Coordinator forklifts out 20 Nurses/Doctors (**cases**), who were observers.

Data collected from (written notes), is entered into a computer by a **data input-er.**

The Chief Whip King fish (Doctor) - in his Salmon Suit, pink stripes, was radio controlled in from native North Canada - for example.

He Specializes in Examination of comparison of notes. This man acts as the (body of Doctor's), makes the final decisions. This man labels us, (corrected pronunciations and **key words**) Asperger freely recite. Words otherwise unaware to us - under less caring formats. (Autistic struggle).

A.S. Spectrum's possess needs (told also - **of**), **corrected terms** we should be using - a comfort blanket gave over; mummy / daddy tuck us up in bed, there, there Son, rest.

You hear a lot of Asperger people telling you we are not accepted via the outside World by and large.

However, you hear never of Asperger saying, his Doctors not accepting him.

Asperger people (take to Doctors) - very well. In my case too well. Sensitive to say my goodbyes.

The Asperger people are awkward in a World where NT.s (Neuro typicals), tell them **they are weird.**

You will never see Autistic Spectrum Disorderlies, of my distinction feel awkward around his Doctor, because it is **his Family.**

A Doctor (GP), encourages the Spectrum Disorder, whereas an outside bustling (Work Force type World) doesn't.

Chapter 4.

Job Centre & things.

24th Feb, 2014 arrived - The day of my work focused interview, with Lisa my Personal Adviser.

I noticed her desk was not in the same place it was from a last work-focused- interview, back Oct 4th 2013.

I walked in the horrible green Job Centre. Job Centre smells.

I said I am here for my 11:45am meeting with Lisa, a Personal Adviser to me.

The guy had to check me out. In his half quarterly joking authority manner, stigmatic of Job Centre plus Employees. He wasn't sure what I was there for till I practically made him aware. Paperwork waving him my identification, carried in rucksack falling out my top Zip, banded by double width Elastic bands. Paperwork orderly - when not flustered.

Eventually I got the famous nod; he was nice today this guard. Said, take a seat pointing me compassed - his stern body language - back further end Job-Centre building I am led.

I sat there with a '**cap on**', glasses, a goatee beard, extra rough sideburns, I must have looked a right odd one - **yet too fit in.** You almost fall under pretences where you are lesser than the act, obliged of your original following self.

So sort of develop a telepathic sort of man spread legs thing. Legs apart attitude going on.

I believe most men guises entering Job Centre doors. Professor types - dignitary gentlemen, subjected in a

Job Centre's cold water environments, may find himself also trances enacted bestowing him, lesser than human.

The dignitary man's (status wealth), had he gone into liquidation bankrupt would get no V. I. P - (**his use too**), people pandering him high held yet now Job Centre broken.

Comfortable - I tend be more, wearing unfashionable clothes, slightly scruffy, though smell nice.

Personally I feel more like Simon, in average clothing.

Though comfortable with the clobber I wear, only becomes uncomfortable for myself, by those who feel needs you must look like them - Fashions in latest, an ounce care - I don't share.

I'm aware what considered Odd Clothing is, it's off the register Fashions diminished. So I know the differences, especially when it's pointed out to you, which hurts quietly.

I happily take all this ridicule feeling like a King underneath.

Glasses I'm wearing like your Grand-dad wore back in days of real NHS Glasses. Dark - brown - red caramel - faded rims lighter shades. Pointed - left/right Tops.

I looked I dare say a bit like a cartoon character, taking one last look in Mirror at home, leaving for Job Centre plus, 10mins early - not to be late.

Still sitting down, inside the Job Centre to my left is a Wall Clock. 11:45am it reaches, the time of my appointment - 'then 11:47am' passes.

I see Lisa leave her desk she asks a colleague where Simon was! I was there all along, disguised in hat, glasses, newly grown goatee.

Simon was Camouflaged. The fact I usually go with my step dad, she expected 2 people sitting waiting.

Lisa finally found me, and the Interview starts 2 minutes late.

She's nice Lisa. I can be myself talking to Lisa without the image most Job Centres give you.

That you are forever careful what you are telling them, (like the way a Policeman makes you feel, even though you done nothing wrong.

Or ways shop assistants makes you feel, like a thief in a shop - while you down the shopping lanes - and the **eye's** are on you).

Intentions of (lying) sits not on my agenda, yet you know you can feel disgraced no matter a willingness plans forecast, (you suggest) forward of Job Centre surroundings.

Hide without them finding an acquired information out. Assumed accepted territory **you don't cross** yet 'An Aroused suspicion' feeling they give you Compensates you no brownie points.

We discuss a number of issues.

I told Lisa I had made contact with the 'Lord Mayor' through good friend my sister's (Nassar Kessell), hence friend of mine.

Lisa got most the conversation started. I presided to say what I anticipated! that the Guitar Teacher's Job she was too find me more info out on back in Oct. 4th 2013 was unfortunately (No Go).

She had contacted, I guess, the (Liaising Governing bodies') of a school we agreed upon. What with my Asperger's, and how kids in Schools can be cruel to Teachers sometimes.

Especially my Asperger's leaking.

We both thought it best, as did others I re-strategic my efforts.

I'm not Qualified on Guitar - the same as I am in Carpentry.

So the Guitar Teacher they do find in their School would have the trim beard, red glowing cheeks, briefcase with turn-y teachers handles.

Images you do see.

Trying other Roots, Avenues, Open University.

I browsed **The Open University** databases on my laptop - Acoustic **Guitar Courses** in their Curriculum, in the sense plentiful - easily accessed - were not jumping out at me expectations! fresh spring waters.

The Only (OU) **Music course** available, (provided only) studies Music under a broader whole hat sense.

So studying: basic music literacy, classical composers, music Notation, music history, so on - skirting topics of this ilk, although stimulating and is of my Interest. It wasn't Guitar specific, port holing 'my time' requires I find; a customized **learning order** my area of expertise, Interests I bag.

The **OU** offer only undergrad/post-grad degrees in Music - current climate I researched my curiosity's.

Don't take my (OU) findings as Gospel just reporting my interpreted understandings.

Ideas gaining the Qualifications, (field in Guitar), Open University were not catered specific and look if they were - nothing became apparent.

I went a stage further pursuing clarity - so emailing the OU's general enquiries (contact email) they responded:

Dear Mr Newell. Thank you for your email. The Open University as a distance learning course provider, provides theoretical music courses as you may have found on our website. Unfortunately we do not offer a course heavily dedicated to the subject of 'Acoustic Guitar.'

You may want to contact a local college or run an Internet search of Acoustic Guitar Courses in your Area. If you need any further assistance then please contact Student Recruitment. Yours Sincerely Molly Greenwood. (Student Recruitment).

The OU were very helpful - contacting me well within their (2 Day) promise answering Emails.

The OU were very friendly - just a shame they don't offer (Acoustic Guitar Courses). I shall return to (Open Uni later), as their (Music Course Modules) they do offer still appeals.

The (OU Music department - in 2014) was rated one of the best in the Country I read, though again I felt much (based a direction towards) Orchestral festivals BBC media music exploring. Again of Interest to me yet not my Order of Importance. Correct learning path, essential when I tailor specified steps on route, benefiting my growth as a Musician not skipping out Courses of Basic foundations - simply because I am well versed myself. The point is I require Certificates so going back (Entry levels) isn't necessarily going back.

I am (information hungry) man; so you can imagine my own frustrations.

Their fees (Credits system) - is in the thousands, so thanks but no thanks at the moment Open University.

Hopefully OU can adapt Acoustic Guitar Modules later upon new designs built in, extra robust Acoustic Guitar theory/practice-laced strong material.

Under grad/post grad - student Courses with Open University, gaining the relevant degrees keyed to my palette, requires certain ((**Entry Levels**)) lower level courses in the (**RGF**) Regulated Qualifications Framework).

Graded 1 to 8 or lower; than those Entry Level Certificates. (Is where I shall now focus).

Again I couldn't find a **Guitar Course** lower than (Under grad/post grad) at the (OU - **Open Uni**), so I will have to think re-think in terms simple, and gain the specific **Entry Level requirements** as when I know - what OU say this Is, then I will be better positioned pointing flags. Armoured Info.

I searched hard a good few hours on the Internet, time days free, seeing finding **courses On-line** I could take.

Gain recognized qualification in Guitar, in Music.

And with my self-taught knowledge I had more than a head start.

Specific areas in Specialized paths, (of your chosen **instrument**), is in no sense (**of order**) foundations to the Top - you could easily say, start here - finish here.

Autistic myself I was looking for a neat, in order list, (of degree specific 'gradings'), neatly stacked from 'low to high' degrees in order.

Yet to understand where to start, and where to finish, was anyone's guess I found, unless you had a mountain of time, in reading through pages upon pages, strengths (the degrees benefited you), where you made a start, where they might lead in reward.

Led by me to believe, you just pick a (degree to obtain), and move with it, no order fashion just pick and learn, learning as you go, not in an order, all agree is the correct order. Him who is blessed with freedoms permissions adapt a free working reign allowances him - direct quicker progress.

Music is an Art, and so where you alone decide to start In & finish, (finish in respect I mean, that Music & Art has no ending, just infinite resting points), before you make the decisions to push your boat, in the daunting, expanding out choppy seas of Music. In new direction you keep up strengths required of dedication, Key Music areas you layout - your own Music plan.

This is why the difference in Music to Art, is an array of different beautiful **start**ing and **finish**ing entrances and exits, in continued learning forever.

So yes will do some good, some bad, where they/you choose ((cut the pie)).

Starting your feed here then growing musically to a Musician embraced, by Musicianship you are to date is again only futures you control, steer murky waters delight.

London seems (place home), of good Music study,

travelling 20 to 70 miles from my home in (Hampshire and Surrey) - unless finding a College/Uni institution closer, with same approved standards.

I personally felt Colleges like L.C.C.M. Or any College dealing with Music in England, in a persons chosen Instrument, they sustain play, colleges like Trinity College London.

All Colleges higher educations under England's hat should allow flexibility's in how Music exams be run via - extra government people power backings.

So with this said, taking Exams On-line, over a set period of time, should be the trend set I believe, or handed down powers you study at a Hall - Church - building - open harvest free study near you.

OK you lack a real life situation in the classroom, yet what with popping in a jam C.D, downloaded software, or Materials of study already possessed in your possession wasting away, then resourceful you works.

Play along - bands persons soloists - DVDs, Blue Rays tech you use, playing as your Accompaniment, Rhythm or lead guitar, horn section, or drums, you see the picture, what more would you need.

Technology allows us to think out the box, that's why we are gifted to take the advantages given. Yet often led by governing entity's pulling cords, not us.

One such College did offer On-line Guitar courses, where you may gain a recognized qualification such as (The London College of Music), however upon the small study I read upon, it noted you must first have at least one qualification in Guitar Music, before you're set free with them. Plus a starting fee £265, eventually leading into thousands of pounds, upon gaining, furthering your experience, higher or extra qualifications, reinforcing already obtained certificates.

I felt it ridiculous I can take legitimately a course I ((can't afford)) by said powers - to show a good **ACTION PLAN** with my Job Centre Plus.

Yet saving money in all areas - by using the God gifted (Materials in Books D.v.d.s CDs already in my possession) - is said wrongful cause I am not actively looking for work.

Study materials in Acoustic Guitar as my subject of following, provided catered by I, on what you tell a College are your (weak and strong areas), personal to you, is you alone 'best judge' studies in Key areas, you are lagging behind or in-front.

As well as outside structures of learning, from Colleges & Universities, outside influence pulled In, tapped into.

The colleges themselves (Music colleges), should provide study materials, within study / exams on demand, moreover they set for you, on criteria asked preferences in an Order you Work alone; born free of payment - your effort willingness to learn is a driven magnet only you establish your rules via respect - for questioning, wastes extra valuable time missing you avoid.

Start Basics in Guitar and or Music, versatile path suiting you better. Modules under your own selection. You may say, well hey this happens already across the Education system. What I am saying is it's a great system yes, and hey, why change (in place) working curricula, greased running on excellence? However, super excellence runs on you building Modules with all inclusive (Study gathering) organized Work your way; 'that is my Way'. Compiled Modules mapped on urgency the (Order) you predict a next necessity they follow thumb nailed - for Music is a 'subject reliant' on swap and change juggling of Informations, where each Individual constantly jigsaw, tests a next move at Home/College, or hey, the back Garden on a Sunny day.

Helps create the freedoms you run with, (ask for), setting my Aspergic mind in clock time, the patterns I can't move or change away from, deny - simply for reasons I have already outlined.

These are my conditions should you want my genuine performance run in Orchestra, this should always be set as your top priority presidents, when help is what you are said providing, with good intentions to a mind of Asperger's Syndrome.

This focused help relates in real friendship, we turn over as a friend. Relations grow, not fought struggles, not ever challenged.

How fast you Study and pass Exams, (is on going), you as a Student, have to be the Examiner in a Way, for you Qualify yourself, telling yourself, I reached a point of no return, now give me my Exam papers.

You start Foundational - Undergraduate - in Guitar.

Have your course tailored, areas of study, you tell your college, you're moving into. Even if your already a real good player, go in as an underdog, never too proud to let new learning (guide), enter and mix with an older learning you come from, throughout all you do.

Through good communications with the college in question, setting the On-line Courses.

You do not require, movement dictated at fast rates, just to rates of study you tell your college your institution is comfortable, before moving staying on boundary pushing, a communication not always universal A.S.

Study materials from Basics to Intermediate to Advanced shall be learned when you ask for Sub-subjects in Music and Guitar.

An (Exam in a Course) taken up via you, taken out like neat folders sub- sectioned, from the colleges Archives, can have the appropriate Studies/ Exams taken in each; (in my case), Guitar - Music Course. Then Certificated Awarded, through the post.

Awarded to say, (you have completed), a certain component, (in my case) learning of Guitar / Music.

You collect these Certificates 'as and when', Study Learned, is Study ticked, energy you are entrusted to freely inhabit, the mind tools of the concentrated mind, a must needed silence to the performance levels you push worked hard disciplines, disciplined you.

Exams on Study taken place, has been assessed, by you

only, or some one of stature, you may further (your markings). Should you be allowed to firstly choose, fitting in time frames loosely or strictly, is again free mind Autistic.

What I am saying is (you), make a Subject Interesting, breaking down Subjects within Subjects. Sub-Subjects.

Having one Student Study '1 week or 8 years' within theory in practices, guideline he masters (pushes himself), him who knows (his passion). Demanding he demanded, it is then him who'll want a knuckling under, rewards he expects set of himself.

Exams taken on Study you absorb.

Fun ways - learning systems, Educations as I describe you, builds an Interest quicker A.S.

Thus more - moreover, you don't require to leave Home, qualifying chosen fields you are building In.

Sense of freedom, movement not told you must be here/ be there meeting deadlines, not requiring you travel further than where you exist, breathe free.

The human heart isn't adapt enough taking short comings the opposite way around, 'pot' your balcony Window flowers, watering watching them grow, (time preparation given). Lump in your throat, successful person, manager of applied thought, put to good use, circular heart circumcised, stepping back staring ages in admiration, all Articulations freely sprouting roots.

I would like see systems I mention take off, so Qualifying you quicker, in baby steps at unhurried sensible timings.

Sub-Courses upon each Subject task in Guitar/Music. Pulled out with as much lengthy detailed mind power on the sliding scale - to simple kept, nothing more asked of you than your own empathy.

Shown orders - firstly logged by the Chief Music Lecturers. Then by you.

Type in communicate - from home on laptop, contact your

local Chief Music Lecturer, Guitar tutors, on your own chosen Instrument.

The Course folders you wish Study this week, Examined in later. Signing On-line (each Course you pull-out), as you would a Petition.

Then what do you know, Bob's your Uncle, granted freedom authorized, by like minded thinkers, Studying these miniature courses, expertly designed fabricated (to maximize, music growth).

In the set out, Music Professors - best stages to follow path. To where he is leading you, or Music tells you, a certain order, required best learn.

Obtaining, the knowledge you build develop grow.

Not all Colleges - Access to learning Courses are the same, nor want them same same ... we don't.

I know there are good systems (in place in Education) Circles - far and wide, this is not my dispute.

Teaching, how they teach, shall vary from a little to huge gaps from one college to another Institute, boundaries same class subject.

So let this continue, dispute your ideas matched on your own mixing palette. For myself it's differences we have, seen from - College to College, from

(Home Studies) - a system rigged your way - to grow your way - to choose your way - granted freedom.

Dependent on where you study, this builds us as human beings, the variety Music remains exciting dictates, resonates rub shoulders, the vast Genres of Music, separates merges, unknown exciting ways, since predictability doesn't give Music, honest listening satisfied pleasure, of substance.

Compared lessons, compared notes, in how we differ helps colleges come together. In what works best. And may I say, great way meet others, journey of life.

I myself am a free-style Guitarist, off the cuff Music.

This isn't taught in a classroom, since I made the Music my own. Dedicated free mind. This is me.

Resonating free Asperger's protects, free bird, help all - who think in such terms, and why I get to philosophize, with less hassle attached.

Music can be taught to a degree, the majority of hard work must come from an interested class, an Interested person, loves Theory Philosophizing as much as I.

The Order, the exercises I give my students, would have started from Fundamental Basics, before I scared them with my Theories, a Qualified Guitar Teacher, cannot be taught, as I am a research based philosopher, stubborn non disputes existing.

It is an expression from Theory head to fingers, resounding out on all 6 strings, you leave with your students, that is qualification enough.

So they have then 'the Guitar Skills'. You grow, you reshaping, re-challenging you forever.

Bouncing Information off, from student to student back to Teacher, strengthens you strengthens student. The Teacher, is not so hard faced, over the moon, when a student is teaching (him Guitar). So a game of student is teacher, (where I deduce in size), fun Music was always meant live, this way messaged.

After a Basic concept of Guitar is taught, I proceed to teach Intermediate Guitar, then Advanced Guitar, for the well adapt, well versatile students, learning as I am Teaching.

Not afraid learning from (your Student), 'knowledge he obtained', I have never seen the likes of.

That is what Guitar and life is about...you buckle, you give way.

Not having to be the best always, it lets your Music Breathe, shows your Students the teacher is human, therefore fallible to make mistakes.

I am 41 to 43 years old - Theory's, Practical Guitar

I was stooped in advanced in, rusted when government stopped my theory.

Studying - I was once... 12 to 14 hours per day, back days in a Labour Government.

To do well through life you 'forgive' blow your own Trumpet, an only sure way little head way provides.

Look pleased, content glad whilst making your mistakes is my advice good, share happy individuality from you, separation that makes you - You.

My Music knowledge performance kept hitting new peaks.

Then when my days lost the 9 to 14 years of hard studying (I put In), I was fortified In to date.

8 to 14 hour days, both Theory/Practical studies, 'put In' must be maintained regularly. Particularly in a subject like Music (Guitar).

Felt worthless piece of garbage, with the Welfare image, Society hated - it is assumed.

My Guitar life took a punishment, through studies hard I came to obtain.

I was on welfare I work best alone, Voluntary manner, seen good entrusted Theorizing for man's better gain. No matter a hiccup system telling us, autistic A.S thinking (does pertain)! set out rules by the lawmakers detailing - '**not us**' (**strains** we work too), Interests theirs.

The days of my study guitar diminished to 2 to 3 hour per days, down further, 1 hour here and there.

They were getting people (back into work), which is good the average person thinks. Tearing up my one only true Interest, I cared about.

Now I'm not expecting a bunch of Roses here, Violins playing for my sympathy's.

However, like when other people already had their chosen Careers in life, they put in the hard hours, an agreement of minds. I told them I work this way, in a greener stranger way.

My happiness for their happiness was not happiness for my happiness, shown back to me, wronged me, stepped on my tail, fore thinking like an A.S.

To be truthful not so long ago, I wasn't aware of what a taxpayer was, in the extreme sense others do strictly.

My Asperger mind worked-out (a taxpayer - was), could quite easily have been a name - given a person who gazumped your house, for all I knew.

OK hands up, I might of known it wasn't gazumping, so gazumping emphasizes point made, so hey Gazumped.

The pressures on my 10yrs of Guitar Theory Practical playing, were to be screwed up - small piece of paper. 10 years aim waste paper basket.

Told ways taken time in a tuning myself, Theory's of Guitar, 'built up long in the making', just **let go** walk away from. All Inbuilt in me allowed to 'rain rust.'

Like buying a new Woodworking Machine costing you £10,000 pounds, allowing slow diminish under people naively blind folded to what I see, nor would they hand me a can of W.D.40 human ways, you thought fought unchallenged original 1st 'Rights.'

Losing the built up Guitar Theory's obtained through dedication, willingness to learn. I took responsibility's for Aspergic - not believing (Work is a Root that suits all), I continued with my Guitar studies, till Government had such a grip on me, I was rusting badly, losing blood flows Interested.

Head of Government, telling you what Right and Wrong is. What a good Abiding Citizen should look like role models on.

Rewarded are those 'whom work Hard' yet denying the hard work my A.S. mind showed potential, showed effort.

They laid out the Standards 'the gov' cut off speech that is me, (whilst losing lessening) creation standing, the creation that makes me - Me.

I worked hard - **work laid out**, I have set out, freedom my payment Credit scoring World. I had worked hard (with seen proof), seen believe follows win over. Denied I find 'debilitating' no seat at the square table. Upset a little. Yet a follower of Jesus I Smile.

So today I looked out my Window, while the World Cup is/was On, I see a bunch of Lads dropping beer bottles in Hedges, time effort required for hired hands, from Agency's some Public sectors of Work, clean up after them, hence more money forked out, by the employer paying the employees. But hey silly me what am I thinking, you gain more Tax paid to you this way, extra jobs established in thine making.

So hey why not everyone just drop loads of Beer Bottles everywhere, do us all a Justice.

I'd love be this Law abiding Citizen, deep down this is who I am, yet when '**I** the **A.S**' left with examples considered bad behaviour, hard in government followed **lessens** me neither! 'understanding'. When they themselves, find tackling such issues, as littering seen going on, in our Roads Streets witnessed.

What happened to C.C.T. V. Surveillance equipment installed in all Roads Streets in England, you got the technology true, not using forgetting to turn on.

Here's another example of Bad Behaviour I personally noticed 'more so I' with my heightened A.S. than another, without living obscurities of A.S.

So here's what I'm talking about.

I Noticed an increasing number of people Harking back, Coughing conjuring back, commonly known as 'Flem 'or (Phlegm, Spit), from the back of their throats.

Seems like a trend '**in thing**' ill-mannered craze, for an acceptance of disturbing wrongs 'this divides people' brought up the **said correct way**, (what we are calling normal) right & wrongs, you as a good mannered person, were brought up to know.

This disturbing intrusive behaviour I speak of is simply

animal like.

Something with as much disgust to me, personally encourages no smile freely dis-taste disposed on you, makes me feel awkward in receipt to their company.

It is, dare I say it very disturbing 'listen too - watch', more so aspergic attitudes - I fight high to stay.

To be '**in**' with the **Crowd**, rub along, frightened to do anything but is wrongful.

So follow in their footsteps (by them setting the examples), we follow in weakness. So doing, is then spread to others in a message 'that they' 'them who' once were polite good mannered, are now, unwittingly pressurized in **copying cat**, those who regard the rules, in what's the ((new cool)), unnatural right.

Chapter 5.

Back to Job centre. Voluntary.

I left with Lisa, my Personal Adviser (Job-centre), copy of my 1st Book, *Asperger's Ready for Battle. The Plain Truth*. Signed.

I asked Lisa if writing books in the future is another way I can Volunteer my time to helping out with Asperger's in Books – I write.

Including writing Guitar Theory Books a 2nd idea backed up, permissions granted. Ideas depending books sought sincerely.

Also away in Volunteering my services to the Government, ((earning my benefits faithfully backed)), not loyally trapped.

Maybe one clear day nothing but the aeroplanes sounding brightening the blue skies, I can pick up a can of WD40, sprayed ((on my rusted out Rained)), Government setbacks. This way 10 years of study is not lost wasted. Man hours I gave of purpose.

Understood Volunteer's Nature, my life will be generating on batteries, ((that work best for my radio)), sign my agreement over to Government the Job Centres.

Should an acceptance "go from red light", green light acceptance. Petrol in my car runs best on dream customs.

At my Job interview today, I have made aware – so Lisa knows, ((all my Books I make profits selling)), are given straight to Charity. Discussing with my chosen Charity's appropriate times, head around ways go about this.

((The Solent MS Therapy Centre Charity)). To no avail. No communication made – no further connection.

So I was forced re challenge myself, look other options, ((when one charity is not a comfort blanket)), my outstretched arm gave.

I can give my profits to awareness of A.S. Helping our A.S friends of non communication verbal. Taking on your charity considerations.

My Banks Manager says I can set up "**Special Charity account**", all Cheques made payable to:

Mr Simon R. Newell. Collected Book sells.

Charity's (advertise – helping myself), Aspergic Autistic thinkers, ((thinking as I do)).

Helps M.S. Sufferer's, all Charity's I subscribe, care to bring forward, so seen as doing good my energy used.

You deny less good coming (from one purchase my books), this benefits at least 2 Charity's Causes – followed below:

((1. Asperger's. 2. M.S. 3. Flood sea defences)).

Giving away (my Profits made on book sells) results I give to Charities, yet damned I am by the elite figures (**in power**) – for not contributing **Income Tax** the business for profit I could easily run accordance.

The Environment Agency firms dealing in Aqua rubber Solutions, maybe where a money's energy is best thrown, ((talking Flood Sea Defences)). Were wait and see.

Pointers suggestions you throw lights on "who to contact." Where best to donate, gratefully receive expand work with.

70% profits as a rough rough guide, from book sells achieved, shall stay left in my bank account, for undecided charity's, when clearer sign post is reached.

Shall stay put, until a presentation day is agreed between myself, the peoples chosen charity books raised.

Leaving me a remainder roughly 30% to buy up Books in Batch amounts of say ((100 at a time)), from my Book Publisher, depicting on how well marketing my books finds resonance forecasts.

Lisa will call me back 2 weeks time Job Centre, this Charitable forecast I lay (I will yes mention) – is it 1stly OK. 2ndly fair.

She can't see this as a problem from early indications, as I'm helping out for example. I will be required to by law sign a declaration, "to the agreed proposals".

The same as my 1st book has been signed over in declaration, the fairness that's sought after.

I am here In making no profits from sells of Books, my bench mark, my promise to you.

However a free reign gives to me, when in the early days I do make profit, used with the intention to root back helpfulness, something your understand later on in my book, without giving the game away.

The Job Centre, for what feels like the 1st time are on my side. Breathing Relief a compromise turned "Corner Stone". Brill.

Job Centres ask me, what I'm doing to look for work. They're not squarely asking me what freedoms, I can exercise into a work, I grow in plans fulfilled in me enterprising.

I'm good at helping organising thinking behind, ((better learning methods)), so why not work with what I am, not interests we discussed I'm not.

Like the Prime Minister, I am passionate, about such issues, so one rule for one, is one rule we can all, promote our dictated positions, angles In.

As are other people Interested, in issues they abstain to – who are: ((Unemployed)). ((Employed)). ((Self Employed)) ((Freelancing)).

You want people back into work, so more tax money, ((is put in governments pot)), then I suggest you find the passion growing in each individual in the unemployment market, so a passion found in the P.M. governing body's alike, is shared.

Happiness in others, should be the Country's, P.M.'s, M.P.'s dream. Should they ask want, ((you be just like them)).

So they are our role models. I must say hands on the table from writing my 1st book, I'm pleased to report governments, are taking a new way thinking seriously, yet how long shall it last?

Look for what an Individual can offer to Society. Go to the extremes of working with him, structures he tells you he wants, his/her – life's go.

I want to work Voluntary so this is seen by me as helping out, "in ways – I tell you", where the work is. I reiterated.

The taxpayer doesn't like Volunteers either, I can only but gather.

Because taxpayers, "are funding Volunteers benefit's still", fore ((Volunteers pay no tax)) now do they.

Yet a good service is provided, by the here Volunteer.

You want Volunteers working in Full time employment right? (As End Goal.)

So Volunteers who want the Full time work capacity, or a multitude of jobs, making up said standard hours, (should then get) assigned an (Employer) his working for Voluntary freely. Jobs matching happiness levels a must.

Each said Volunteer ((who is/works for)) – "this adapted Employer" pays taxes to the government, eating away responsibility ((track a Tax)) from the Volunteers, new adapted ((Employers)).

The (Volunteer's Employer), has always gotten a great deal past history gone. After all he's not paying a Wage to Volunteers, as has the case been so many a years.

Also no Employer ((pays no – Volunteer's Taxes)), the

good work we do freely, which should be claimed by the government helps keep the deficit down, promotes newer better ways to juggle an already over complicated Tax system, in the free cleaner universally accepted powers, battled through parliament. Thus more, it promotes a man free willing.

Making past "**free work**" an Employer once was getting from ((said – non tax paying – Volunteers)), Employers should pay "the taxes" ((a Volunteer owes)) – said to owe.

Since the Volunteer is working (for him freely), disadvantaged his kind soul, cannot pay tax, so is he a benefit cheat for this reason !

The good (Service) provided, our Volunteers give to all namely Organizations Corporations firms, termed his Employer, should, I believe do what's right and pay this man's Voluntary Tax.

You can argue this wrong, but when the ideas I speak of grow wealth in the Governments annual turnover of Taxes collected, then what better way to stack a claim. Furthermore, you won't have to Tax your Bank hungry friends so heavily, or nip into their bankers bonus.

The Volunteer is still getting benefits, yes for sure, but then you can argue, he is working for his benefit now, much like he'd work for an Employer, had this route been more appealing, but now working in a capacity that the claimant's (mind works). So less Mental health.

And has all the labels of benefit dodger, duck & diver, released from his soul.

So if the government start saying, OK every Volunteer in the Country today is seen as helping out, earning his benefits justly "Announced over a loud speaker."

Saying: Full time Volunteers/Full time people in Work, seen both now as equal fair approaches, a person's life choices, chooses this side of the path or this divide.

The ((Work carried out in both cases)), Full time Voluntary, or In Full Employment, both get the same Jobs done in life, it's just who pays you, who pays who.

Where the source of the money is coming from that ends up in your pocket – his, hers, their, is the lifestyle you are better worked In, for your asked for set Conditions, and shall have you divided again, ((**in the person you are**)), ((will continue as some losing out some winning)). Therefore, what should you do? Well, what you do is set a pilot scheme up, run the scheme, then flaw it, should rehearsal not win realities – true hand.

The real problem it seems, they have – ((The Government)) seen through my eyes gaining Fungus, it's already Fungus.

Yes, a Volunteer can now be seen as working for his benefit, from the unemployed person on benefits, he was before.

So thumbs up this is good right? Nope, wrong. Why?

Because the Volunteer, although climbed a notch from unemployed earning his benefit, is presented with another problem, through eyes the way he'd interpret, suspect the government would see it.

That problem is what Simon?

The Volunteer is not putting money in the pot in a form ((government seen taxes)), that some shall Scream shout is Unfair. Yet rehearse this pilot scheme previously talked over. Organizations/Employers, paying for their hired Volunteer worker's Taxes, then it's job done.

Volunteers helping out in communities these guys. Voluntary benefits ((he is paid still)), by government from taxes. Is collected by other people ((paying In)) that ((do get paid)), who do pay taxes in full time work. So tell me, him whom receives a Wage to him voluntary man not asking Wages – tuned his way, has only his efforts rewarded by them whom call him a scrounger, a lower life.

Paying out Tax to ((Unemployables and Volunteers)) telling them they're wrong, yet not collecting a Tax from the ((Volunteers Employer)) so we can wave a banner clean is unjust – please review.

Giving ((Full time Workers their due respect)), you can't completely disrespect this angle of thought, so is not a wrong way to be, may I add. This is just one element of tactics seen as a Good person and Law abiding Citizen.

The other tactics elements, I Simon talk about is the Good Law abiding Citizen I try be, with the way my brain works under the Umbrella of A.S Autistic.

And why a good percentage of my elements making a case ((are loopholes you look for under review)), when you shouldn't. You should accept a man's way he shows you a help, when I address them with an honest Tongue a fair man understands.

I don't wish too rub any of my aftershave theory the Way I Philosophize "on over to you" if a sternly you were already not feeling or rigging to the Justice good, my boat is chugging swimmingly.

My argument is this: I the Volunteer see my Employer, ((as the Job Centre)) or Organisation firm benefiting from worked freedoms I centre must follow. However ridiculous this rubs your shoulders, the other way, is still a perspective of thought I can't change, since it makes sense to this person me.

The Job Centre is an organization, same as a Work place an ordinary person attends. Is organization firm based, both these organizations pay money out to people who are helping out working for them.

The only difference is political issues, people see as fair or unfair. To the source of money, where each uses and questions, so pay people who work for you. ((Without paying them discontent)).

You might say well TAX payers reluctantly pay Job Centres to pay people who are Unemployed or Voluntary. Stacked argument in-use I'd guess as a come back answer. I only imagine from my source.

Well OK, sure TAX payers pay for (other people), but the

big butt is this, TAX Payers are also given money for the Work he does, from the Employer he works for whoever this is. ((So that is – given money)).

Volunteers are (given money) so I see any difference you argue as a 2 sided road equal. Furthermore, I accept your debated arguments caring enough I drop the debate split the road, walk on happy smiling.

And where does the Full Time Workers Employer rake in his money?

I tell you where ((from people who are Volunteers)), willing to do something for free. Money comes in from many many sources, from the Employer's Customers and Clients. Right down to the factory floor.

Money motivates people, but those who work freely are motivated and help out by dropping money as Important, yet are blamed cause they pay no Taxes.

The great emphasis is wrong in this World. Tax payers wearing the arm of justice one sided law. This Is a Country strangle-held choices sucked right out.

So do you see, there's good arguments on both sides of the fence, a lot I've not covered to keep your boredom down.

It just comes down in the end, what family party you support. Support your ideals just comes down to how your brain is wired, that sees truths and lies, unequal good bad in all at varying degrees.

Arguments only waste time over debating, so the way I see it Aspergically ((is – just get on with it)), don't think, don't question others, just accept that's how they are wired.

Or feel free to question. However, just remember stay prepared, ((he/I'm)) not going to lose running truths I run with.

Money that could be funding other things, other than paying one more found on benefits Volunteering, who by the way is helping out with good intentions, could be argued by me Simon, that ((TAX payers Money, a person receives)), as long as you're not spending it on Drugs Cigarettes, Alcohol, swanning it down the drain, using the money you felt you earned through Volunteering or good intentions by Saving it, maybe going self employed with this Money, to do the right thing, so you're seen as a (fair contributor), is yet more of the arguments, that may come face to face with you.

Yes Simon, you can twist the truth around many ways, although one truth is true, it don't stop another truth, from being true either.

Sacrifices where ever made will always still leave some moaning, even when we (give in ways), to (please – them only), leaving us disappointed. Us being the think out the box people.

You end up with many truths to be found, when an honest study is taken, considered honest by you.

Only one truth can be honoured at a time.

Same as you can only put one finger in another's ear at a time. ((Known as a wet willy)), I was informed.

Since there are only ever 2 Ears, listening to One truth, one finger at a time.

The Volunteer owes then really the problem is, ((a tax his duly earned through hard sweat)). Yet he's not duly paid, as he kindly was saying alright, I'll do it for free, which by the way his doing.

Who pays for the Volunteer, for the good work his (given to the community), yet not been paid by an Employer.

The Government/taxpayers pay for the Volunteer unemployed – to do good works, in his community.

Taxes collected pay for ((Public Services)), Volunteers are that Public Service – provided in a multitude of Greener ways to work. So why discriminate?

Is this the Volunteer's fault he prefers working as a Volunteer unemployed, or is a man that can organize his life cleaner, the way his minds works, powered clear acceptance only.

Or that the Employer he's working for as a said Volunteer ((Won't pay him)) – cause he's getting something done for free. ((Something for nothing Employers)).

Why doesn't this ((Volunteers supposed Employer)), his working freely for, Not Step in and say.

Ok, government/taxpayers, ((I'll take it from here)), I'll now **pay my Volunteers**, "for the work" I had gotten done for free in the past.

Cause I didn't or wasn't, ((paying a supposed tax)), the Volunteer "owes", denouncing him as nothing more than a scum bucket, deserves not a denouncement I share In his burden.

And will work with you ((**he says**)), if it's a free choice given to me, (work in free ways), that strikes good heartening blood to my veins, ((cause it's not compulsory I pay)) "it's freely I pay" the working relations ((he – I – The Gov)) – witnessed.

You see what love is your fellow man can do.

This methodicalness seemed deemed right by the here by ((taxpayers & governments)), alike.

So the **Employer** "the Volunteer was working for" freely walks away, has a hard hard think, ((he thinks this)):

Err-rm, OK, well, ((what if I'm to contribute fairly in Society)), in seeing a fair system for all, ((I need to **as the Employer**)), whom has Volunteer/Volunteers, working for me freely up until now take on board enterprising work abilities for all, that benefits all.

And I ((**he says**)).. "as the Volunteer's Employer", pay a tax to the government here on In that they, the Volunteer can't. As the Volunteers branch humanistic pulled weights.

This will in theory make him the Employer "poorer", only slight poorer off scaling **everyday taxpayers** good news ((it will make these guys richer)).

So it's in the Government's best Interest, all taxpayers Interest, ((to find a said Volunteer, a said Employer)), who will pay a **lions share of tax**, for the free services he had gotten for, so long before.

By Volunteers helping out. I think we can agree on, conclude ((Employers still do save money)), **by not Employing** Volunteers **full-time** taken On.

Just Work done freely with a "**slight Tax**," is not going to hurt his pocket, as much as it would, hiring a person full-time, with a full wage to fork out.

This should be sat on heavily by taxpayers/governments alike, if you are saying, it's not fair a Volunteer ((is – **paying no tax**)), but like still helping out.

Stay with me we're almost through.

So look as an Asperger's person myself. I don't care too much about, or take on board "who gets what", or if he pays more taxes than him/her, or Charlie gets 2 chocolates, than Rosemary receives 5 Chocolates, (so that's not fair), yet Charlie's 2 were rambunctiously more Delicious.

One thing learned in life, what makes fair for one person, is something you've not on purpose "but have made" unfair on (another others), sub-sequence to decisions you changed to benefit one, sleeve socks corded.

Like some prime ministers will benefit the Rich over the poor or conversely. Someone always loses out.

Cause eventually you must make a choice decision, that was hard or easy.

For example up until now, taxpayers have been paying for our Volunteers "it is said" in direct, indirect manner of thoughts, mainly through Neuro typical's mindset.

Moneys taken from him the (taxpayer), by the government. Still divided up by the government, through the channels used like optic fibre balls, computers highway sent pay a Volunteer.

Indeed if an Employer of our Volunteers working freely, starts paying a Tax for ((his our – **tax paying friends**)).

Then other tax payers will see it as, that's one less Volunteer – (their outgoing tax is going to).

A feeling of fair play fills the echoed House of Commons. The house where (Bills) new laws are filed through, preparation open speeches easier to build a (**stronger case**) – than time Writing a Book.

So you the government now have more money in your pot ((if one less taxpayer)) or all taxpayers' money has stopped ((channelling down)), into a Volunteer's so called lack of payment, who can't pay his **taxes** – he currently don't, "unemployed's alike" **pockets open.**

Through no fault of our own Aspergics, Unemployeds, ((without Morals matching, some with)), are all thrown in the same barrel, depending on who's in power.

Unbalanced not perfectly symmetrical ((to the face of fairness)), with policies that peel off quicker than a sticky label on a woollen jumper.

The Employer who agrees to pay a – (same Rate of Tax), ((for his own Volunteers to government)), as a same tax others pay. Is contested as a balance of free thinkology – you can't lower as wrong.

Depending on (Annual) you earn a year "to relieve" **other moaning taxpayers**, is more of the battles an asperger like me ((will look)) happy, balancing the scales.

Making him, the (Employer fractionally Poorer), also other Companies that have work done Voluntary, tad poorer. This is again ((some will lose out, some will win)).

So you see – you've certainly done what you thought was right, made others poorer in the process, namely the Volunteers/Employers/Organisations/Corps.

Hex all of Us.

So what's the Solution Simon? There is no Solution, only sucking up.

There is no Solution, ((It's not what you know, it's who you know)), we were told !!

So "what you know", and educating yourself by this message above, is thought very little of ((when you have **no – "who you know"** friends)).

The Ones ((Autism's people)), feathered down to ((Asperg's)), **"don't have"**.

Trouble seeing an A.S. does – "It's **Who** you **know**" as more placed larger importance over **knowledge** to **"what you know"** placed smaller emphasis is more of the battles Asperg's alike will struggle.

It's life's fluctuation in the unpredictable up/down high/low peaks of your life, an asperg can only fully be one with conviction.

Some people get lots of highs, some lots of Lows.

Some a real dolly mixture, so it's the experience we inherit, making us the shaped people we turned, "still turning into", that we work best "in one atonement".

Hope that made a little sense. I'm not here to confuse you, just lay with you my A.S. truths.

Gee Whiz is this dude still talking Voluntary. Sorry yes.

A Volunteer is giving a "**Service**" to Community his outer Society.

Not paid for (his Service) "by an Employer" for he is a giver of free circulation, no matter of tax problems he encounters on this journey.

He rewards himself as doing "achieved good" to how he asks a ((condition of his mind, **be set**)), be met.

With very few bargaining chips at his disposal. Meaning he's automatically boxed into a box, that disables his growth, ((for his good will shown)), to how his larva volcano's "the juices" that gives him the name Simon ((or your name)), persons handicapped in mind freedoms, the same as I, same as you.

I require freedoms like the concert pianist.

So this guy – this brazening Volunteer ((is all his life)), set in a disadvantage background package. Oppressed, he's repressed the skills he offers to the table, if he/they of the same – didn't meet strict timetables, ((of the **Tax strategic savvy**)) that makes him "him."

So he himself may expand in learning, that is of non dictatorship, find an honest world of heart, set in place "as his main" all eggs in one basket focus of interest, all else falls in lines secondly to him ((people of my stance)).

Wronged further when his mind he works with/I work with, is controlled to others' delight, hard line tactics, that he – I am not of "this substance."

Especially when I've logically reasoned through a logic I'm from, no matter how many people come against me to dangle their views "that's ready" to slay the good dragon in me, the clouds of good feelings. I must run with keeping my Interests high, light hearten fun.

The Volunteer is not paid, because he has fairly been paid, ((by the governments' Job Centres)) in a scheme moulded to – modelled on his better working guidelines.

So I say to you softly, if you want taxpayers to not moan, you should target the Employers the Volunteers are working for, something I more than repeated in previous pages. This employer may come also in a form of Organisation/Charity based foundations.

You the government/people in moaning, should expect (Employers) finding cheap labour. Too pay pick up tag, his Volunteers 25% Income Tax (from him), ((to the governments lobster pots)).

The Employer is still getting a fair deal, so is the Organisations of similar roots. He's **not** paying **full wages** out, just 25% of wages **as Tax**, that the Volunteer has fairly earned that he owes – to Gov.

You kill 2 birds with one stone, for (our taxpayer) is now gleaming his happy too.

And the Volunteer gleams in equal appreciations shared.

You still in-hinge extra problems however, even if the World shaped up as fairly, as I have given it to you.

And me taking truth's path with you, whether or not truth is your quest.

Problems alive cruel World, an Asperger shuts down under from, hides under the blankets, pinned down under strain an over-bearing Authority (**must do**).

Must be suited the same to be accepted the same.

No energy cared. Aspergic person playing the game of honesty with you – ((his honesty)) – is often spoken over shut down. World he is joked at by.

The same energy you were asking him do well in earlier (**he give**), not contributing in a seen way, ((you deemed right upon him)), is seen by me as a double edged sword, branching off in many jungles of truth.

The very same people, you are calling fair Tax payers, fair because you the government made it fair. As the compulsory element.

How many of those tax payers, would pay a Tax, given a choice?

Which people in Society would pay you the Government a Tax. Left to an Individual's open house to decide. I'll tell you shall I?

The **honest** in **Quest people** Voluntary, so you the Government distribute fairly to (Services) requiring paying "systems of work" brought around, soft caring workers, hollowing the name, good citizens pay.

Percentages, people whose quest is – not sticking to honesty, but have to by law pay a Tax. From every watched penny they earn. Are the ones.

That make the ones whom want to try be honest of quest – do the considered right thing, **seem wrong.**

Yet by doing so "the right thing".

Having Asperger's what we want to do Is slammed back in our face. Ouch, from ideology's we abide by – our disability of awkwardness.

All the time. We see what makes sense to us. So what I'm saying to you is (if not paying Tax) is a message that's – not fair on others.

And hey it is.

Than me earning money from a person (**employer**), ((who will pay taxes to you, the government)), from **my lion's share.** Cause you yourself said, this is honest in quest. Should out of respect, only have honest in quest people working for him – working for you.

Since asperger people will need a lot of open space, friendly faces where ever he goes, from job to job or town to town.

Having an honest in quest Great Britain is all fine to visualize, makes better for your children to come.

However for those who can't share a vision, you feel the love in, perhaps cause of the up bringing they head. The age they are now. Or you can't teach an old dog new tricks.

Pulling up now on your Harley Davidson's, come along "and say" Hi, we the Conservatives are your new honest in quests.

Only now have half-baked honest inquests turned up, through hardship peers led in him before.

It's a taught thing in Society, it's no real big deal, what the government thinks, so don't bother Voting is a stale message I don't like but must agree openly unfortunately.

Only Asperger – mentally ills Different people use honest quest rules much degrees, work his backside off, to pay a **human Tax** to you one made of knowledge, not metal coins.

Not eliminating – people, going against the grain like me Asperger's Autism ((Disabled handicapped in thinking this way)), ways I pat myself on the back should, I believe be Government's top priority.

Better formulas ((to his mind/my mind)), I/he was given of free speech once, free will. Christian heritage, a God caring people ((if more money)), is to cream its way into the Government's lobster pots, they take pride back rewards.

Since loving your neighbour must be a message ringing in not just 98% people requires love 100%. So do Asperger people.

For their head knowledge please (not toppled) – not stop no more.

With the A.S. means working with their "sensitive ways", diligently not rushed, all the time in the World, yet progressing a World you turn around to his love, helps helped his progression.

Loving your neighbour as one such Principle helps the ((right from wrong messages)), we are told about, built differently in others, all people it may seem.

This Is one such principle, that requires maintenance.

So our Right from Wrong Principles, don't mixed up along life's bumpy rides.

Chapter 6.

Here's a list of things people say as Neuro Typicals "I avoid."

Thus putting huge space in-between me and those I Avoid.

Reading my Case studies: Aspergic cousins may side my 1st views. Or simply find he is different than me. So I share my Story.

Literature - emails scrolled back - fourth gingerly browsed, I confirmed (my own diagnosis suspicions) 'after'. Seeking to find A.S Knowledge low level curiosity's others of my Condition bore was not born Interest I cared quick info compile. I had Asperger's and looked no further outwards, I told my own story.

Before I was clarifying similarity 'I firstly only knew my own symptoms'.

This all suggested too me, sort of people my cousins were A.S may side; share experiences add bonus Identity different they want away from me Individual A.S flair something Special the many Shapes A.S cuisine on excellence.

We're far more disquietly profound, than my non-seeking self 1st virgin mind suspected.

A parallel tangent thus running concurrent isn't - Waves only crash illogical.

So here is a rough guide: people may on the Spectrum mostly Avoid 'I Avoid' found in me.

1. People who say: ((Who is He?)), where has he come from? Like they were the 1st ones there, when we were understood, we are here for reasons we knew about.

Our Autistic friends may happen to find the! ((Who's he)) people, (in a place), we hadn't asked them to be "either."

Yet were friendly as all people should, our awkwardness showing, we can't breathe the same air. Our heart irregular not open as it should remain.

In a meeting of strangers, 'around us then', we have no idea why they are here either. Those who we A.S. Happen to find, are in this same place.

At a place & time throughout life, you're made awkward for being in this same place, yet we had good reasons purposes, 'to tell you' what the Nature of our Business was.

We didn't ask them be there, much like they didn't us, vice versa. However we turned up with a friendly nature that's instilled within us. They obviously (stance) - for being in a place where we turned up too - ((we have no problem with this)), we just wish sometimes people were, dare I say gentler.

((Them, and we)), 'stay on this side, the other side', of the Fields - divided uncomfortably.

These same ((Who is He?)) people, gain supports from their peers, by saying ((Who is He?)), and they sit there, like they are, King Arthur.

Eating their Overly-sized Chicken Drum Sticks from the K.F.C. around the corner.

Like we are there for the Sole purpose of their Entertainment.

We Asperger people may have a 'Meltdown' lose our rag - stick together saying, no Sunbeam friend this your actions is our wrong, worded with A.S pattern quietly in our shadow walk away with more added uncomfortable mental feelings we carry home, our (goodwill) - honed we were wronged In.

2. The people that say: 'How did I ever meet you, people', when most the time it's them who approached us seeking a friendship, we had no regard for. Though being the friendly soft touches A.S are known for, we let them in our life, for the experience, then later wished we hadn't.

I have left you space on numbers 3. 4.

And more (numbering notes) - you may jot down / add separate sheets notes, for you remembering your uncomfortable situations, or you'll have to have. Always avoiding if when possible, places you walk cause you're showing good nature - apparently wrong.

3.

4.

Here's now a list: of people Asperger's get Close too.

1. Families.

2. Love guided **friendships.**

3. Sensitive freedom **types.**

4. Winning of **heart people,** not winning of economic prosperity.

5. Glowing an **energy** meant of what **you see glowing people,** not anger mentally reducing us people.

6. Joining people, people you're able to almost say anything around, without **step toeing walking on nails.**

Arr you may work out a few for yourself. I leave: 7. 8. numbers blank.

7.

8.

Chapter 7.

Book Mistakes. Hans Asperger's.

When you make a start writing your own book 'your 1st book', will be real Good.

You will have above standard story-line, you will leave the story running. Tidying up, with a darning needle, ((not all holes)).

You will want to see some of your Jumper's story, with a little thread showing. In-fact you will want to leave in your 1st book, big holes in your jumper, not repairing or caring.

You are sewing as you go, (losing the ability treading every crack the pavement is offering, 'so not perfect portrait'), weeds growing of mistakes. Put simply in a new wording, it's impossible to fix every pothole in Great Britain, so you accept the human element in your book, or your always be, (held up at the train station of mistakes), without advancing your free motion that is you, so letting mistakes grow in you, 'twist vines in you' is encouraged by I.

For example my 1st Book was left with purpose, you not finding 'neat Chapters - headings - sub contexts', good presentation demands. So cause demanded has me swimming a freedom (rambled) - not to show off, staying nobleman. Instead broken up/down Autistic bombarded, so the high class may snigger laying in simple effective ground works.

I recall (Elvis Presley) was subjected to **well to do** (people's sniggers) In films I watched, so maybe people only love you when you make (The big time).

By doing this exercising, it allows extra freedoms in

future books (the Author takes on), playing simple/ complex writings introduced, both or just irregular uses, the mind identity you push for freedoms relaxed.

You will leave your 1st Book uneven (as a book), all books started out this way.

Later you may bring out re-edited Revised Editions, of books that horrified you, given another chance to spin perfected interests breathing your real voice, selling your books the added pound extra, to previous underdog limelights you traced an outline sketch.

It is a shame the old Victorian wooden beams, ((be sand blasted)), In your books, loved to a perfect world ticket pleasing far too many - you see.

'Split lines, In Victorian Beams', strong bent over nails corroding, with those amazing, ((Horse Brass Ornaments, some laid into a leather black backing)).

That Victorian feel beam, taken out your Book original, leaving you without the Country feel it intended.

Even the pulled threads, in your jumper's book, you will leave. Small & large mistakes your book has, is eating away at your own Spiritual fabric.

The human mind likes to see a clean house, with the Air Freshener gotten out once in more than a while. However a too clean house, shows not the mistakes your book, rotted with Wood Worm ran a love.

A Clean Palace gave you no experience, since you never made no mistakes. You hid put a drain hole cover over mistakes, ironed them out with a little starch. Sprayed them up in the old man's garage, your Grandad's.

People stepped over the mistake drain hole covers in your book, at least those nurturing mistakes as loved new baby's, or cradling a cat in your arms, reassuring mistake makers, roads too genius. Just don't go hating the 'ugly in you'.

All your books lived as a crisp perfection - (had you wished) which is not wrong, however your Crisp Master

Piece, doesn't happen till you're on your 8th to 10th Book.

15 to 20 years have passed you by. Shape-shifting clouds your life passing, you wrote magnificently 8 to 10 Books.

This is more than mission Accomplished, nevertheless your books all 8 of them please should work like a 14 step staircase.

Each book, showing a 10% increase betterment, to the One gone before. The reason for this is, you are showing you are human. And when you are receiving your medals on the red carpet, you will feel very relaxed with the evenings presentations.

8 books however of perfection made you too crisp clean Author, therefore you had to walk around the rest of the evening, with a dirty big smile on one's face.

The humanity elements in your 8 Books had you left the mistakes, still at your evenings Presentation. Gave you a power to slip off the shoes, laces too tightly tied, slippers on feel at home, holly-wood feel factor.

Now people are coming up to you, with those flute champagne wine like glasses, saying Simon my good fellow, can you explain the mistakes you left.

It opens up a door, whilst wiping my banquet dinner misplacement's with my napkin, you suckered your audience in, waiting twitches on the fishing-line, in bite expectancy's you set up - a truthful answer you found easy, then gave.

All of the manhole covers in your book, were stacked up left open.

And the evening continued.

The evening's guests at presentation night fell down every single manhole, cause all mistakes had to be explained. Only fine answers cackled approvals.

Aspergeric people don't like explaining, so they set the traps book tighter than a tripwire, then cur-boom you captured your guests.

And wherefore you do explain in whistling a cloth through their ears.

Ear suction they now do hear better.

The crisp clean 8 Books at the night's Book awards, had no guests asking you no questions. Because you had made no mistakes.

You were instead walking around the Albert-hall, a statue of perfect, congratulated in wrong reasonings. The award ceremony took place, I felt out of place disjointed, (missing my mistake friends), yet thundering my own high command to prove a point.

The problem was you were being someone your book wasn't allowing. Everyone else was chatting away, knowing you had Asperger's, you'd not allow yourself, go up too another in starting a few words off.

Questioned in private conversations you put in great performances beforehand, tied feet no matter my good advances.

You with your Asperger's expected all your guests to form circles around you, the A.S. thinking I am acclimatized believing, loves universal traction.

Why should I bring my 1st steps forward going up to someone else. You were N.T thinking. I was A.S thinking

Problem is the whole Albert-hall thinks as so. As a new face, you need really get out there, making them sacrifices.

Reach out your hand, that has built up a sweat in your pocket - (the hour it stayed).

Clean the sweat, when no one's looking, say hello I'm Simon R Newell Author: Asperger's Ready for Battle Plain Truth.

With new books on way, like babies born without 'Reading Glasses'.

You will feel better showing yourself as A.S, not an A.S. (Some might pretend they're not).

You met a new lady who took an interest in you at the presentation night, she scribbled her telephone number on your hand.

You lost the (clean crisp image) you went in with firstly earlier at presentations.

You instead used the image of mistakes, and lost & won fought topical debates all night.

The new Aspergic Simon was re-born known as the Aspergic norm.

Taking on much strength writing books, realising when walking out away from your writings, no one else sees the voice (you), they just see a stranger who's walking past them. A man 'out and about' in say ASDA just a regular guy.

Talking of mistakes.

My 1st Book I said! - ((Hans Asperger)) who discovered Asperger's I assumed was German.

It actually turns out he was (German by name), more or less, 'not Origin'.

He was '**Austrian** in **Origin**'. So I do apologize.

No one has pulled me for it yet, like the traffic mistakes policeman.

It's just nice to know I can loosen my tie, pop a top button, knowing it's OK to have a book resting with mistakes, not having to know all, remember all.

It is easy critiquing a Book sitting in an easy chair. So remember as hard as perfection must keep your wheel alignment digit point zero; the human Author is not word perfect I am A.S.

Just make sure though I stress, that made Zero tolerance when you're dealing with ((Factual Mistakes)).

Should you make One Factual Mistake as yes I did.

Don't then try phoning up your Publisher, asking for a

quick mistake to be rectified. As this is not giving the mistake come mistakes an allowance to breathe, let it niggle away at you.

Chapter 8.

I Joined the Army.

I joined the Army at 17 I believe, it wasn't the Regular Army (Full-time), I was a Reservist.

I was a real TA Soldier ((Territorial Army)) a.k.a. (Territorial Force 1908 to 20) (**T.A.** Territorial Army 19**20** to **67**)

(TAVR. Territorial Army Volunteer Reserve 1967 - 82).

Name: ((**T.A.** Territorial Army)) was revived in 19**82.**

More recently known as: ((Army Reserve)) present day).

I simply prefer to call this reservist volunteer group (TA Territorial Army). There's something of tradition in this name humanistic. Re-branding the name to (Army Reserve) feels for my concern heartless, a sense of loss.

The year was 1989, my memory serving me correct. I was enrolled it felt like, in late Spring to Early Summer.

'I was introduced' when I came Into Army life, Into ((Intake 5)).

I had only been out of School a year, when I think back. Though I felt older, and was still very Immature.

Though Immature outside the TA gates, I threw my Immature Simon 'in my Bergen,' ((Huge rucksack used by Army Forces)), acting out my 2nd role.

And mature Simon, would be seen by other people in my ((Intake 5)), New World. (Stepping into Uniform, from Civilian Clothing), persons who joined up at the same time as me.

I guess through my life, I'm seen as a different persons, (people). To the different personas I use in disguise, in Camouflage.

The Nature of who Simon is. Cause I'm not sure who he is at times, through being different people persona to different people. Helped me discover who I was, unafraid to be hated or liked.

I was.

The Army TA Centre was based in Stanhope Rd.

Commercial Road Portsmouth, named the Connaught Drill Hall.

We were the: 2nd Wessex Regiment. 2nd Battalion. A Company (A Coy). (Duke of Connaught's).

This Regiment was broken down into 3 Platoons. I was in '3 Platoon' - Infantryman.

Thursday nights were Drill Nights, used generally as get togethers to discuss take debriefings, future events planned On what and if we went away Weekends. Including physical exercise/weapons training, and much more presides.

A breakdown of 'Weekend events' voiced by our Sergeant Major and (Colour Sergeants) the overall objectives. As a Unit: talking too all 3 Platoons knitted together, as One Regiment One Family.

Then after our Sergeant Major started the night's proceedings, (in our overview talk through s...), we scuttled down to lower ranks: Sergeant, Corporal, Lance Corps for further debriefings.

Which was very Important. You tuned in carefully, to what was being said spreading around us, or you'd miss out on knowing what it is you should be doing.

Nothing worse, asking your colleague, army buddys, what 4x4 Lorry am I on again, what platoon am I joining, when arrived at Reading Barracks for example 'am I in.'

Bit like peering over on a School friend seated next to

you, paper textbook his cause you didn't listen to what information currently circulated around you ((from the off start)). Asking people reluctantly what information you didn't grasp, others may make you look small, ((for not doing so)).

So a responsibility was built in each Army recruit individual to tune In, listen up.

That's why we had Thursday Night Drill Hall Nights so you would know, (have a picture in your head), where you are breaking down movements yours, instructions clear, the Weekend's away - ahead.

One Thursday night Private Darren Brown turned up at the ((Drill Hall)) and! Also in 3 Platoon army colleague, ((had made up)) at a T-Shirt shop place, inside Commercial Road of Portsmouth.

20 or so - 2 Dozen, Hand printed T-Shirts. They were Red with black lettering.

Can't remember precise design picture, was roughly a machine gun with crossed weaponry design.

Though something I do remember the words - spelled out:

*((Three Platoon Take No Sh*t)).*

It was great we had T-Shirt empowerment the other 2 Platoons had yet not thought of, walking around the ((Drill hall - Mess halls -)) Pubs Bar, upstairs 1st level, all in Connaught Drill Hall.

In our - (new designer Logo T-Shirts). Rubbed the other 2 Platoons - feathers, I dare say.

That's the Competition you must have in your Family Unit, Regiment.

This creates a movement in lifting the guys' Spirits to try do better than us, out do us, to keep Momentum up and Moral High.

Secretly all though the 3 Platoons in our Unit were seen as - 3 different Family's. We were One Family in actual fact under One roof, we were just too proud to admit this; is all.

3 Platoon consisted of: Myself, Corporal John Weston, recruited Introduced me to Army life; he worked as Carpenter & Joiner in my Apprenticeship days at A.E. Hadley Shop fitter's, Hilsea. Portsmouth based firm.

He recruited me worthwhile (thinking Interest) about joining TA Army, as he see I enjoyed fitness, noting I had bags of energy. I took on board John's talks while working at Hadley Shopfitter's and joined.

As well as John and me we had: Private Mark Ray, Private Steve West-Thomas apart of 3 platoon.

Private Agar - although he might have been from another Platoon.

Corporal Dave Prodger - I loved this person he was one of gentler helpful Corporals. Everyone bonded with him, (he hated no one) apart of family 3 platoon.

There was another Corporal, Kev to his friends or Kevin, Scottish small guy, hard.

Nice man, long as you fell in lines followed tasks out given. Corporal Kevin Caden. Corporal Caden too us Privates. Again 3 platoon material.

Sergeant Steve Barwis was 3 platoons Sergeant among other duties including P.T.I. Instructor - you know white vest, red rimmed.

Jack Rafferty also Sergeant in 3 Platoon. Happy soul always smiling, real army spirited one of the guys.

Neil Baker was our Platoons Officer addressed as Sir, Saluted in appropriate places.

These 2 Sergeants along with the Platoon's Officer Neil, Mr Baker to you & I. Were more of the glue of 3 Platoon, who made 3 Platoon what it was.

Good strong Characters - strong sense of Humours, needed when all plonked in same Boat, told to work as a Unit.

A personal respect, went within 3 Platoon, to our Generals & Officers in Command.

Intake 5 was now complete. We were 1989s **3 Platoon.**

There were undoubted other Privates, and higher rank others filling out 3 Platoons bulk I just cannot remember all, fore 3 Platoon was reshaping & remoulding always often throughout my 1 and a half to 2 years I was In the Army.

Pinpointing our ever-changing, sometimes not changing Platoon, Is Hard in giving the details Precise.

Sergeant Jones, otherwise known as Ginger Jones to his friends, joined 3 Platoon in my Career, he was more of the Glue 3 Platoon required.

He had the makings of what 3 Platoon were looking for.

He was English/French, had Served in the Regular Army, The French Foreign Legion. Hard, you wouldn't want to mess with Ginger, but one of the nicest people I've met.

Corporal Onions joined our 3 Platoon family for a spell, he reminded me of Keith Lemon (Comedian, Entertainer, Celeb, host). He had elements of Keith Lemon residing in him. No, I'm not a Keith Lemon Fan, but Onions was liked, I liked him.

I just got worried about Corporal Onions though, as on a Weekend away, we were on a (piss up) with the lads, he got on stage in the function hall we were in, can't remember where we were.

Though one thing I won't forget, was he proceeded to eat a pair of pants, soaked in his Pint of Beer, cut into strips from the long hard weekend he endured away with us.

He was now eating his underwear. Animal hard to the core.

We were wondering if he was slightly Warped, but as time passed us we realised the man was just one of the boys, and so loved his strange ways.

Most the time Onions was on the Level. Very intelligent man part of the Signals unit army, drafted into 3 Platoon.

This was all going on at a time I hadn't been diagnosed with Asperger's. One because I don't believe I had Asperger's then, I was once ((one of you)), the Normal people. Dormant AS was there though sure, no one questioned my difference seen, no one had a name categorizing me as Autistic. In them days it was a nicer World, a spotted fish would not seem out of place - nor did I.

I'm a Special person with Asperger memories of Normal days. In Army, Schools, Colleges, home life.

'And two' my Asperger's character I'd yet to take on later, hadn't had the finger of extraction prodded highlighted on it, only transparency blank. Back in time, there was something a miss yes, (I knew this) something that made me stand out from many, though the World was a very different place then.

Doctors - lawmakers - people in general all ordinary people families those frozen days everlasting - periods of time, language survived on good naivety blessed innocence. You never worried about tomorrow, life was forever open skies the air was godly free gasping honest my lungs carried. I walked forever alive forever you required no thinking beads beyond difficulty. Complete wholesome we weren't questioned we were understood. Energy of brown & orange70s. You felt like you could Speak say anything the breath of fresh Air was the World we Walked.

17 years old around close age, the way I was shackled hope in my moulds, must have gone by very quietly, my diagnosis had gone under the Radar, or put simply, I was accepted for the character, I threw to others, they thought I was. An invisible diagnosis not seen in me yet.

I Visited the Lord Mayor.

I visited the Lord Mayor of Portsmouth recently. Ms Lynne Stagg. (early In 2014). I Mentioned early on.

My visit was led in conjunction with my 1st book. I sort of knew my first book was no great seller so I simply handed Lynne a signed copy, and enjoyed her attention gazed hands by my side. She began ask me questions .

Lynne said Simon? why was you only diagnosed as A.S Autistic. Say 10 - 12 years back.

Good question Lynne! back previous to my discovered (diagnosis) I mix with people once better than I can now. Though saying so, I walked the same lonely path. I find happiness in today's Day my diagnosis had no magic white line this side capable Normal Simon, then upon diagnosis discovery, suited up as Simon Autistic. It just was not like this at all.

Although I felt my diagnosis more under awareness, self conscience now (my thinking) can have an explanation. I had to be Special in life from early birth to this typed word. My diagnosis signals all Autistic people (fight) when, others tend (impose change on us) from conditioned Special.

I had to show I was strong if you like covering up how weak I might of felt.

In my early days, running full Backpack weights equivalence near 50 House Bricks or more wasn't unusual.

Running from Hilsea (area in Portsmouth) a loop around a Mapped Circuit. Heads South towards areas (Northend. Fratton. Southsea. Eastney) - outside edges of Portsmouth cut in my runs inwards where suiting - 10 to 12 mile runs. Finishing drained back at Hilsea. Gatcombe Park. My home.

Running bigger circuits, on a Saturday, or Sunday depending on other events cropping up.

3 Miles at least every single Night.

Maybe Lynne indicates my best Answer I may leave as my explanation - why my diagnosis Asperger's remained invisible.

In a World brought up shown; loves white soft blue energies.

Life in (my first half), triggered happiness and so granted, disguised my own open susceptible self.

My diagnosis is brought on more seen, when my raised way I developed as a child (developed inside loving settings) is ignored on political correctness pressures, AS don't work like this nor do I.

If you had taken away this friendly love I functioned normal In. Then opening a ((clam)) opens my Asperger's no empathy.

Clive's Shed.

Along with this 'training running' I did for the Army, I was Weightlifting with my friend Clive Thornton from Hadley Shopfitter's, professional Polisher by trade. (Every other day - 2 hours after work).

Scheduling training sessions altered a lot. Both me Clive had separate life's, we spread ourselves thinly.

Day to day things were 'played by ear' cancelling postponing, should one or both us not make the dedicated time slots, moods not swinging a Rhythm today.

I loved Clive, he helped me grow get (big). I was becoming a solid puffed up statue of a man body beautiful twirl flex. He wanted a partner to go to the Body Building Competitions he Involved himself in. It was a nice thought but like it didn't pan out as so.

I was more Happy Body Building myself in Clive's Shed after work.

His wife would call out - 2 or 3 times, bringing us away from the Shed, cool down healing, a cup of tea and a naughty cigarette for example.

She made us laugh, she would purposely put Clive off ((his Rhythm he'd built up)), bench pressing.

I'm not familiar with Weights we lifted, today in 2014. But I think it was like, (20kg 2 weights) - on one side, 2 weights right-side the same. Adding decreasing weights the exercises forward unfolding.

Depending on the Exercises we incurred, be it Bench pressed, standing up with a Curling Bar, Dumb Bells, e.t.c.

Squats, behind the neck lift 10, front above the head lift 10.

Clive's lady sometimes put Clive off in flow pumped up training, a feather between the legs maybe, or breaking his serious train of thought. Making him laugh whilst on his 14th lift Bench pressing, trying to push out his 2 last lifts, arms slowing shack trembling.

Lips making splayed, gritting teeth, trying not too laugh.

A fart escaping. Oops uncontrolled. Bending, thrusting our limbs working it hard.

Me behind him ((Spotting)) for Clive, to intervene & assist Clive should he signal me with his eyes. Spasm arms locked, push. Rrrrr. Push one more Clive - good enough rest.

The Weights used changed in accordance to Exercises we scheduled planned Routines.

Clive's Shed was his den. A get away from his wife. It smelt of Body Building, old brickwork. Chalk marked repetitions, lifting belts hung up, smeary windows, private dwellings not to disturb. Set back end of gardens reach. The sweats we fought through years, with me, and personal training Clive did for himself on his own.

Weights were everywhere in Clive's Shed. Big weights, rusted weights, new weights, different colour weights, Iron weights, plastic weights. Believe me variety was there.

I was Confident in those days. I was a Virgin to what was going on in the World. I had no brains. I thought everyone loved, the same as I do.

I thought every thought, passing the Chalice in my mind, was a Wavelength all people used.

My Army life was helped by Clive's training. He wasn't in the same Army as I. Clive was a P.T. Instructor Army years ago.

You see Clive was 36 at the time, I was 17 to 19. Army in my blood.

Our age gap changed no love in our friendship, it was the day we were in, ((that was the same age)). We trained in Spirit as the same age. Locked in the same day. I'm now 41, 42, 43, 44, when this Book publishes.

Clive I lost contact with. He would be around 58 to 60 today in 2014. If only I knew where my good friend was...?

Memories is where he is Simon. Thanks for that Clive.

Asperger's - in the now and before.

This book is entitled Asperger's, so I better get back on track with you. It's also entitled Simon's Normal life before Asperger's, so your forgive excuse my interludes.

It's Asperger's you are Interested in though, is why you took your copy off shelf. What you must realize is a good percentage of the Autistic Spectrum are Diagnosed 'not straight away'.

Therefore, you are asking to see the Dividing lines, before diagnosis, and after.

If Asperger's, the after diagnosis is your only care, you're not then seeing the Diagnosed patient in 2 lights.

You are seeing him only as Asperger through, through and through. One life time only.

Back to the Lord Mayor, Lynne says Simon, Why were you not diagnosed before?

I knew the answer, I just couldn't give her what she was looking for straight away. I had to walk away from the Mayor's chambers.

Pose this very Question she asked me on 17th Feb 14, to myself, when I could answer with sincerity.

The answer wasn't coming to me straight when I wanted. Same as you don't always get what you want life modelled to your 1st decrees, before working hard efforts, reach high jobs, higher answers establish.

Not always getting the answer you thought you might.

In visiting a Clairvoyant, the Spirits don't just come through because, (you paid £20 to see a Psychic lady). Money is not the dominator. Though through absent healing, the answer may visit you in holy spirit status.

When the Spirits - levels, 'are ready to come through' to you, not before.

The reason, I was not diagnosed in 'Early Stages', personal believe mine, (I had no Asperger's in early years), or at least not an AS you could see.

I became Aspergeric studied when, age had toll on me, is a theory I work with.

Though in my ever-changing Asperger mind, theories are changing when (Spirits give new answers), new advances advises.

I listen to my conscience for answers, our Father (Jesus/God) Holy Spirit, ready to show a confused answer, to now shown clear reasoning.

Another theory I uttered, is it's quite possible I had Asperger's in my quote, Normal days, though the Asperger in me was laid dormant. Thus hard detect appointed Doctor in times way with me, not seeing Aspergeric tendencies.

As an Aspergic person I hold true. Asperger's is a worsening condition as the studied patient, is getting older.

Don't shoot me down for my theories, they are my theories.

You can quite easy screw up theories I've laid to bare with you, like Scrunched up paper. Listen to other people as well.

Or you can listen to what your heart's theory (says your theory's are).

I was Active young boy, as a Normal lad.

Knew there was something very different about me, Special if you will please. My sexual side thoughts of habit, let down my good side in life. At a 30% sexual/70% Good ratio. I had part sick suggestive devil thoughts. Sinned as a result wilfully, holding thoughts not contemporary. From the 1970s climatically developed child, controls movements in Union. I knew right from wrong and am not afraid to say I am a Sinner.

I know looking back (perfection is not me), just strove purification. Thoughts were wrong I had, with weaknesses in me, but they did happen, they did occur, nothing can change that.

So yes, in what I thought were my Normal years.

In that yes, I joined the Army. I completed 3 and half year apprenticeship, under the guided wing of Hadley Shopfitters. I won Apprentice of the Year.

Was weight training with Clive.

Living in Bournemouth on block release College, which was part of the agreed apprenticeship rules. 22 to 24 weeks away from home - per one year, purposely unevenly distributed each consecutive year. Learning skills, growing with my carpentry tools knowledge in college.

Return home train journey, back in Portsmouth from Bournemouth college to Hadley's work place my firm, I was with in apprenticeship.

Skills obtained in College, put into practice in ((Work real life situations)), for say a belt of 30 to 28 weeks a year in Work. Again broken up in groups, uneven blocks, consecutively spread set out on timetables.

These block releases at college and back home with Hadley's: ((22 - 24 college)) - ((30 - 28 work)) weeks to no not exact formats.

Were - in timetables, so through circles year, it would surprise fluctuated timing.

Break this down further then. Example I was at college ((5 weeks one Block)), back home at Work for say ((7 Block weeks)).

Back to College for lets say, I don't know ((4 weeks)), back at Home for say ((3 week block)).

So I wasn't away at college solid, totalling 22 weeks.

Was split up in groups of say (5 to 8 Block releases) per year. All Incurring (different block lengths - weeks) timings, spent in college/ spent time back home, Work Hadley's.

Staggered uneven different timetables from point A starting Apprenticeship, Ending my Apprenticeship. 3 years 6 months complete training undergone.

Shining in many Persona's to different groups of people.

Something that can't be **calculated** to the **many changes** of **faces - I am. I was.**

And so with all this Hive of activity going on in my younger years (I'd say I was normal), problem is my Asperger's wasn't born yet. The nicer World it was in 70's 1980's showed a clean teeth diagnosis normal.

My Diagnosis was not inherently seen in me yet, and if it was, fun laughter a loving World disguised cotton wool normality, my Asperger's could survive green nets camouflaged thought of as normal.

Traits requiring an association to tie me in, as One thing or another is more pronounced when considered normal. Autistics are not permissioned to show their normal ways they best function.

Autistic ways seen within me in my early staged days (yes seen), yet lying dormant like Cancer, no one banded hurried a name to my said normal sided Simon, cancerous Asperger yet too develop.

Softly I'm asked why was I not diagnosed found Aspergic - way back when.

The Doctors of the time, was not the same World as it is today. It was friendlier, less Political correctness had to be achieved. People knew I was different back in the day & now. Yet to be diagnosed AS there isn't always a doctor on every street corner handing out free pull up a seat checks, on stall. AS like before the turn of AIDS in the 80s, was not in public affairs public communication, talked about very little.

They just didn't have a label yet. No one was tapping me on the shoulder whilst I was lifting logs for the army. Army (log runs) at: 06:00 hrs mornings, saying hey Simon we are calling you In, cause we're keeping tabs on your weird behaviour.

Therefore if I was showing (an oddness), it certainly wasn't in Army time.

I was a weirdness to others I can appreciate this regarding my difference I'm displayed, going to shops yes. Other activities, general busybody clash bumping open public strangers, friends, family's familiar, Hello dear, fancy meeting you here. My conduct normal walking alone, now altered strong Autistic mixed communication my startled normal self dissolved.

I was showing a weirdness in my apprenticeship at Work yes, yet not at College - not around Army life.

I was 2 very different people, in the walks of my Apprenticeship. From the split transit of: Work/College.

So the strong, well-liked person I was in the Army, which was my part time job. Was given opposite the Cold Shoulder by some in my Work Environment (as Carpenter), who didn't know of my popularity in my Weekend Warrior faced hive of activities away at Weekends.

Simon was seen not known to have a job - in part time Army. No one at Work knew I was Soldier.

I guess my brain couldn't separate a clear line of ((having to be - liked everywhere)), some places I was liked, lapping up bonds made regarding being the same liked person. Other areas of my life meant I needed a separation, to relieve the other Simon growing in me well liked.

I still wanted the same amount of friendship good luck

loved crunched in, yet at my own price - my own pace variation accepted in me, liked on merits mine.

I wanted to find other Rhythms my Drum differently drummed, ((experiencing the same loved received, I wanted no matter how I was banging my Drum)). Yet receiving hatred & love all at different rates, so I could keep an open mind not caring whether loved, hated, disliked. I just required to show both sides of a Simon growing deep cut pains.

I didn't mean no harm showing both sides of me. I just wished I was loved in equal measures, not frameworks I'm - liked in only. Naively I believed you should love expanded exercising light heartening soulful me freedoms. I had to work this way.

I found I wanted to be a person, sensitive egg shell stepping diverse with, ruthless in openness - as well. Still be the same liked person I was places I was liked loved before, it wasn't enough to be starved in one persona of my character, I had many ready for exercising.

I felt I wanted an instant just like me will you.

All the while still wanting to have love/liked given the same.

With my friendly, ruthlessly odd openness, as the new price, restraining my energy wasn't easy. I instead showed an intelligence which came out as Silliness, cause that's how I coped with vast amounts of Information. However people weren't taking to my Silliness I found a release in me, helping me.

I wanted to be liked/loved for all reasons liked/loved in all Places, such as the Army, such as at College. If love's compounds were about loving the many shapes, an ever changing sometimes not, my human way.

Sure I understood why my Silliness wasn't liked, wasn't approved. Reminded often with snarling looks beady-eye staring of discontent, huffing stand-offish, cause it would have annoyed me the same, had I seen someone dancing around the same.

Yet I confer - I still needed this 'Silly boy Image - I was', for the help was given me faster learning I set better healthier fun love not given - had I showed expected Normal Ways.

How could I show as Normal before or after my diagnosis - I'm Aspergic right? - Well yes, just wish others knew and I knew, back days then earlier.

10p Coffees.

They just see the Apprenticeship boy buying in coffees for the older boys. Going to the (works store) asking me to bring them back - 100 quarter inch holes.

Or a Bucket of Steam, or Stripy Paint. Whatever the lads jokes were at the time I fell for.

I was known as Chocolate head. Dave Robbins, our machinist, lovely man named me so, cause I would eat a good 10, 12, 14 Chocolate bars a day. Sometimes more, depend really. People thought I was confident, hard maybe overly, yet only so after my chocolate fix.

Eating chocolate gave me a temporary rush. I needed comfort.

Looking back, I should have been a lot more focused than I was, in Work. I know the bosses only with reluctant; vindicated my absolved me. I got away with a lot in Hadley's looking back, cause I was young a boy who knew of little no better.

I had a very playful Nature. Would wonder around the factory floor talking to people, whilst Ken Carter/ Alf Cole's - (A.E. Hadley's foreman), spotted seats in the look out tower a.k.a (foreman's office). 360 degree vision situated half/ half sandwiched in both 'Machinist' between 'Assembly bench - areas'. Like Mongolia poached egg visioned in middle, Russia, China surrounding. I kept a look out for the foreman, when they were away on business calling them - not to be spotted drifting away from my Bench, where work was set out for me, on scaled drawings: 1 to 5. 1 to 10. 1 to 20. You name it e.t.c - scaled drawings actual sized drawings (scaled down) - to fit on paper.

The paper they used was of a professional tracing paper kind, regarding Scaled drawings. Used I guess for ease of use, unrolling on overly-cluttered benches of the Carpenter previous job's wood shavings saw dust.

I put all my efforts in gaining respect being liked as a Person, when I was in College, in the Territorial Army only mainly, you've heard me say. This meant I sort of dispatched less gave up. Gave myself a break so not trying as hard at Work in Hadley's (the images held of me) in them circumnavigated my first impressions last (up held) did not.

And even if I could turnaround my first impressions last - image, and had I done so, my survival fights you see, 'not this perfect image', I am Simon, open.

I felt there were 2 Simon's/3 Simon's/ 4. Numbers of Simon not remaining static. I was as 2 different Simon's seen I'm sure and more, to the One Simon more Simon's - everyone thought was the One Only Simon spread as across the board.

Which in Normal thinking terms is correct to be One Simon as your collective Self. Though my Oneness was only achieved ((as Asperger)), when all my collective selves were liked to form the One Simon.

Liking all my (collective selves) - adapting my changing as and when I needed to reformulate - ((was not respected was not liked)). So I keep a wardrobe working out which each individual each group likes - and give them one Simon only tasted to suit on osmosis. What they receive is fake Simon. Partial Simon. Losing Interest rapidly Simon. Symptoms referring me back - locked in Syndrome, my own World A.S.

It's really a matter of perspective, and how you see things, but being A.S., no matter what you're seeing, how you're mustering, I believe loving the many perspective combinations we are, to how you said, ((you only liked this Simon)), is not enough. I want as general a bit more Stimulation than this, I want more pound for Ruble.

Letting myself down in Work. ((The Work place)), showing

others the Silly Simon shall we say, as Simon No 2 to my persona.

Or (Simon 1) sensible white collar suited - if you believe I'm Simon 1. Shown to all others, general perceptive - of well-liked me regrettably only ever knows, others seeing (what I showed) this Simon to full well be - in turn famously the crying shame.

I guess for everything I was 70% good at, ((I needed a solid break)), so pretending to this 30% of people, to be the let down Simon - for my sanctuary comfort their despising my sought rest. Yes it hurt me, but I still needed this break. Being what everyone wanted me to be was (I was liked - as long as:) I shopped at, spent money at their store - voted their party - fitted into such a clique it was cliquey as hell. You don't have private healthcare then you're NHS scum - your personality the person I carry myself as - means your earning potential is less, ridiculed under my hungers.

Although I was Simon No 1 in College, the respected try hard Simon, about half - 2 thirds of people in College see me as odd **(not the Teachers).** If that's the right way to express.

What was going on here in classroom sitting down - and practical classes. 'I shone Teachers favourite it would appear' - disliked keen energy I displayed. I walked a tightrope happy learning, losing friends college buddies meant I was for my money on track.

The air in college with the Students I was placed with, gave me the signals as such, the space separating us.

Don't get me wrong, all my college colleagues were good soulful people - they liked me (with distance) - as I did them.

I didn't care really, I just wanted to do well, grab my City & Guilds Qualifications in (Shopfitting). Then get out of there. If I had to put up with a few disapprovals, not mixing - no big deal, bring it on.

So I did **Gain Qualifications** in the chosen **Career path** I chose.

And so I did obtain my City & Guilds in Shop fitting.

Getting think it was a: ((**Pass**)), a ((**Credit**)), & ((**One Distinction**)).

Ok wasn't the Highest marks taken from College, from our 12 or more strong class Shopfitters, but who cares. It was more than satisfactory.

I think I done well at college. Well in the fact I had an eagerness to want to learn, should meant ignoring rest of the Class, sat in the front rows, really no skin off my nose. Yes did it.

The dropped comments from other students I could not leave 'unparalleled'; my direction for them born Autistic.

Cause I showed them I was strong, I showed them, I'm someone who knuckles down, when I'm not disturbed. Directional Condition concentration my A.S. led me.

Giving my other college student colleagues their due - on the same course as me, they did I must praise them, 'let me get on' when I showed a discipline. (I had to work) as Simon lonely, yet Simon approaches A.S. - my take on things.

Army & College running side by side.

Army life - College life. Slightly staggered when each started/ended. Though for our bulk/main body, they were paralleled together - 'main bulk of time'.

I was in the Army at the time of College. I was finding the overload College work assignments requiring my homework brain, throwing on a Pair of Size 8's at the Weekend was/were - over lapping each over.

College was seen as more Important, as too Army.

Since it is the college work I was doing, that was setting me a path my chosen Career at the time.

And so yes, had to come 1st In front of my Army life, upsetting (turning my back) to Army. Giving **one up** had to **go.**

I loved Soldiering. It's was where my daydreams were going in doodling college lapses daydreamers pencil.

Eventually I had a word in Mr Bakers **Ear**, my Officer 'above me' 3 Platoon T. A.

Explain in wordings I practised 'Mirror' the night before to get it right, on the day.

I am sorry Neil - I mean Mr Baker Sir. My Army Career is overlapping - into

College. I must give One up.

He took it like he understood.

Showing no weakness he was sorry to see me go, I knew I would be missed. Cause I had same Emotion running through me, for all my Comrades.

Things hurt in life to let go of, often same things call things, heighten our bettering Success we are told. Not just because told, because intuitive from obvious assumptions not spoke. I could declare this rang all true, just wish I hadn't felt so guilty, soft emotional.

I went home, packed up my (standard issue Kit bag), all recruits are given on joining up.

My dad's army helmet standard issue, which most my army colleagues (exchanged in buying them-self the **Kevlar Helmets**) later. They looked better, weighed less.

My hairy Mary army shirts, 2set Lightweight trousers, 2pair Camouflage trousers, Webbing, Ammunition Pouches, Kidney Pouches, 2 Jackets camouflaged with all the pockets, Mesh Tins, Leather boots Parade/Field, Trouser Belts Field/Parade, Beret cap badge, the full Char-bang.

I didn't want to give my (Army kit) - back but everything I wore, **was government owned.** Including my mind at times. Though if you've ever heard the saying ((we're tough - but we're fair)), well stick a label on here with those prints. Cause like that's the truth an Army life, stuck family matters strong loving each person as a person (was what mattered) body of men.

No Good for you my boy.

My Mum felt, Army life did me no good, in so many words. I don't think she meant on first sounds.

Meant distinctively more so I think, that is when my drug habit fitted a same time space.

Meaning she thought it was timing from point A, I began Army life, to other side, See-saw point B, my Army career ending in time.

Of a Look back 25-27 years ago I was in the Army.

Understand I do see why mum, link my Army life, Drug life, run concurrent. Links together.

Less Army, my drug life took hold - no link I remember. I was naive happy spirited making lots of Army buddies. Army gave me good energy.

So naive I was 'of the Workings, of this World' I was an easy prey. And was - (a supposed army buddy), who asked me for my telephone number, just before after leaving the army, whom was in 2 Platoon or 1 Platoon.

He freely Vaseline's pure naivety my clean developed mind, real baby's bottle weaning me onto a new word, spliff I'd not heard of. Here I was with a rather large cone shape in my hand.

Mums link 'see drugs affecting', so most people Normal were correct 'links in' same vein of Army, untrue though on my first take on things. Sitting down thoughts, you'd know both may determine correct and wrong.

To be strictly fair nonetheless, the Army's tolerance on drugs is Zero. Army through my own experience forever promotes only good health, with army friends you hook up with.

I didn't know what Cannabis was.

I seemed to be more naive than most Children my age. I was brought up in a World of cotton wool, shown ((Only)) what Good was. And wouldn't have of wished no upbringing other different. I was very Lucky.

So I was vulnerable, easily led down the garden path. As long as I made concessions in my mind, telling myself this guy is my friend, then I didn't care, I just wanted to be liked. I thought what I was doing was, (having the given love, I was giving to my friend), ((he whom introduced me)), to dare I say the word drugs, was automatically accepted by me through him. Half-truthing myself this guy is giving back on equal paths.

And so hey, I chose to close my ears - believe the truth I pretended I heard, as I set it up in my mind, what I wished to believe.

That I'm not to question, if I'm to carry on feeling the level of friendship pleasure he gave me, I told myself was there. Deep down it was there yet submissive to his kind dominance. It is difficult to tell when a friend is a friend.

I thought good his purpose to my friendship was what I convinced myself whole halfheartedly was there. Yet all along I knew deeply not true the case, carrying on, ((in what I - wanted to be true)) not what was necessarily.

And so my mind was pumped to not question.

Though I felt it was very one sided, I didn't complain.

Was just glad this guy was the friend, I said to myself he was. Wishing looking back, I'd gotten out the friendship sooner.

Honestly you boys.

I'll be honest I didn't know there was bad people in the World. If I did know, then they were the Villains, only Good people were right in my mind.

Although the person who 1st introduced me drugs, was wrong in what he done, I am sure he realizes it now, or has throughout his life. Deep down this person was a Good person too.

And it was 'this sense of goodness' I see in my friend, converged with biker-like badness to his other half. That maybe was why, (I held on to a friendship much longer) than necessary, for the kick in the teeth it done for me.

If you yourself try change someone from bad to good 'you see in them' the bad they use at the tipped forefront - ((then hey do yourself the big favour from me others, you're wasting your own time)).

Their suck you in thanking you for what you see as, you helping them, while nothing you are thanked for is satisfactory long enough. Secretly they despise your good Samaritan tactics, appreciating you enough to build a message of good work drilled 'what they can gain' for what they see as weakness in me in you. That helping gave no more reward than had I not done zip on a cleaned slate untouched for my friend I'm pleasing.

Then without so much as a warning ((spitting you out when you're off your guard)), neatly stacked up thrown back in your face, for good you effort-ed their way, in trying to be the expert good Samaritan. So now you open - your Back Sack Satchel wider, 'Walk it away', hardening yourself vowing never to care for others before yourself from this walked step forward onwards forever ever again.

Is why 'from now on' you put your own welfare 1st, ((knowing you can't help others)). Unless you're showing help to yourself, (the help you wanted to see working in them), as near same good human only limited powers.

Not asking 'others join you same' it's a choice, a glow in you, you readily accept adding to your already wisdom, never trust in people ever again. The way I tried to change 'or was that help people' you think or believe - you can ((save)).

From their wrong/your right paths you see alone. Signalled out by you, the do good-er (you see in others - or he we call 'him') never goes down well by you 'to him' - telling/drawing attention to a considered friend (of what you're about to perhaps denounce perhaps promote in him, as categorically wrong, plain & simple). A voicing to what (right & wrong means to you) '& especially you only' that you after a long, long while point out the 'real you', ((feeling no guilt or shame)) for being yourself, to him the once friend.

This is especially true persons who easily hurt with Asperger's can't voice an inner voice - and why non verbal communication is seen in Asperger's not all roughly - 60/40 split.

Changing ((non - Verbals - to Verbals)) with vice/ versa roles played (does happen) why we are a shell of protection.

Asperger's has learned his lesson never to give help to others again. ((And why when we don't)), we are seen in another bad light. People say why are Asperger's people 'so rude' so quick to turn away.

I was thinking about my good friend who introduced me to drugs ((to myself)). He was probably the same innocent well loved little boy/child, I had grown up in the World to be. In fact I know he was. A following chain he perhaps was changed from once innocence.

His good & bad combination '**was only Good** once upon a time.' Nevertheless under peer pressure, it's a crying shame ((his good in him)), wasn't strong enough in the fight ((he as one grew)), out succeeding the main growth of Good to a good shown shaded.

A shame he had a greyer, shallower side too him like **Darth Vader,** fighting the conflict within him.

I don't want to talk about this person any longer, cause he showed me **55% Good** that's being kind. He gave me more than an equal share of 45% Bad. Dragged me **down,** naivety innocence I started out in life.

You see cause I didn't want to lose his friendship, I still followed him around. Eventually this good person in me (continued) yet left me from angles what (onlookers took), so my Name was dragged through an undergrowth.

I was humiliated, by the tittle tattle, his easy persona breeds new friends. Rendering what uses In me, he found he could perhaps grow quicker up another friend's ladder, now mine slips lesser default wood-wormed thoroughly.

Bringing me down, by displacing me with confident punctures. He left me with many holes. I can't keep up repayments - new puncture repair kits.

Once people build a picture of 'first impressions' last, they also judge quick without seeing the naive person's side to his persona. He certainly made sure every mouth brace was tightened to his designs. That he told the story to others (of who I was) defenceless to perk-up & say otherwise, can be expected Worlds normal A.S walks away from.

My friend was Neuro typical - I was still un diagnosed Autistic, so maybe this unknown diagnosis I was when I was regarded Normal, played in same fields clashed.

Sure I could be strange to others, I had Asperger's right, though I had nothing to put it down too back then. I was just Simon.

And still to this day I see him as a friend when really I am told I should exact anger spilling of my paws.

God told me, you heard me say in 'The Plain Truth', love your enemies Simon. So I now do my best loving them the most.

Though giving my best love, to those who humbled me as friends. Those who radiate Love, with the Intent Growth requires. Real Love you first were told about.

By the growing Family, the parents said World should of been. Disappointed to learn otherwise, each day ticks with slow.

Damaged troubles.

I'd damaged a lot of my Inner circuitry's scarring left with me through drugs, that you might well say could have triggered my dormant laid Asperger's, I didn't know about. In any or either case, it certainly wouldn't have helped in any case.

The person who did all this too me, don't talk to me any

more. I tried staying friends with him, but he didn't want me in his life any more. He'd had his wash with me. The damage he left with me was fulfilled, through jealousy orientated something he felt, he wanted to take from me.

I didn't really want to be a part of his life no more, was angered to let go easily, even with all God's will, ((of God telling me you don't need him Simon)). I was still hurt, the time wasted. I didn't make friends easily because I believed In having only one friend for the rest of my life, so other friends weren't Jealous.

Though was hanging onto something, cause I was now a changed person from the good World mummy & daddy brought me up into, I felt I had something stolen away from me, ((& I wanted it back)).

So I hanged around as the friend. Smiling with an angriness that took 5 years too lose. I was really hurt.

He Loved me all times I was doing things his way. He was a good 7yrs older than me.

And once he said to me I recall, 'you're more of a brother to me Simon', ((than my friend)), who lives only 4 Seconds down the same road he grew up with, all his life.

A neighbour he'd grown up with he'd come to accept, 'it is thought' ((the close friend)), the people who are apart of miracle of childhood-friends, or so told this story goes.

He had the experience to over bowl me ((the friend I talk of)), sliding with thrown on the rubbish heap, when I was no good, or not pandering to his wishes. Like finding a replacement for person's been sacked, there is no shortage you know this, he knew this. Softer persons can't replace friends so easily. I couldn't just abandon one friend for another disposable *Bic* shaver style friend.

That was my taste of our real World how Cruel I found it could be. I never understood why people were like this. I just wanted to be friends with people. Found the best friend, I met was forever myself.

I always use to question myself, why do people get so angry, turn nasty? I just didn't know why the Love I had for the World, wasn't shared in the same Manner.

It just made no sense to me. So I tried seeing myself as people 'in them' (I didn't understand peoples shoes). (And what they must have gone through).

They mustn't have had a good start to life, that I was given by Family 'I born into'.

I think I had to give way in the end - accept. Not all people had a good start to life. Questioned it no further.

Any questions I was asking as to why? I was keeping very personal & private.

My Drug Use wasn't to get No better.

I was introduced to Cannabis at the age of 18. My drug use wasn't to get any better. I had a very addictive personality, clung to people.

I met a lot of good people (who were good), taking drugs Cannabis.

That's all I took Cannabis. 'I say all' yet this was wrong even by buttering up its glory.

I remember all the adverts, with heroin users, other drugs alike e.t.c. That we had the talkings to from our class assembly at School, frightened me enough.

I was not purely of this ilk of Nature, from the get go anyway, (class A) - so I was well protected in my principle palette, to know this is basic fundamental to ground wrong. Out & out.

That even now this day, I'm baffled, puzzled to what looking back ((a fool I was - am)).

One - because I see the affects.

2 because I instinctively knew, felt class A, drugs were wrong.

So although a message of softer drugs leads to harder drugs in spoken word theory and study result statistics, a message stronger spoke in my 70s, 80s, 90s years changing e.t.c., so on, forever.

It's not what happened to me.

I was on my guard with other drugs circulating, avoided them with a stern fist. I never met anyone pushing drugs onto me, it was all above board. ((It was through choice that led to harder drugs)), not from what I experienced in near on 20 years of drugs, a witnessed push.

Real life is far not like in the films. I found it to be much more friendlier controlled, so even though I'm not here to pat drug usage on the back, that's all I will say I experienced to its congratulated effort.

My only claim to experimenting any further, 'was a bad idea', wished I hadn't.

When I took an Acid tab Micro dot, becoming a ball of Energy for 2 to 3 days, that's how long my ((trip)) lasted. It frightened me more than anything, I was not thinking as I should.

((I'll be honest, I was frightened)). One small pill - One millimetre in size, had more power than all Presidents over the Globe, warns you of comparison.

I had a motorbike at the time. I'll never forget the day I thought I was going to die. I just wanted to get off the (trip) - I was currently on.

Once you popped your ((trip)), there's no turning back. Best you do is go with the flow of where 'your trip is taking you.' Colours alive more - a World a body sleeps, walking away you hear sounds inventors on the highest tech equip can't produce comes enters your World. You better be strong Indian chief.

On the trip I was on 'I had a motorbike' I said - at the time of popping my pill, a CB 125 Road bike.

It was only a Provisional Licence on L Plates. This little machine was my excitement, I was only young.

So you can imagine the excitement can't you of telling people you had a motorbike.

Not knowing though I had Asperger's.

I had something though.

I popped my LSD trip in Winstanley Road, Stamshaw, where in a bed-sit I lived.

I had lots of strength, what with the Body Building I was doing. Past tense hobby's also muscle interests in the now.

Couldn't believe taking a little (trip), no bigger than a needle head, ((could do so much)) it's reiterated, very frightening.

Upon taken my trip, I thought maybe 'I'd received a dud.'

I nibbled again one third microdot nothing. 20 mins elapses nothing.

22 ish mins - then no word of lies I started coming up. I was entering a new World fuzzy hearing, new worlds started roll tunnels through my hearing canals mine. If you didn't believe in Jesus 'now was the time to pray.'

I had not no word of lies counted in my head 125 press ups I gave closed knuckles bedroom floor after microdot swallowed. At a young age you might expect I do 50 at a push.

I did not lie 125 push ups.

Scarily hungry for more after 125.

Man oh man I was pumped up red energy.

My body was use to being pumped, the mirror posers of body beautiful.

I than stood up in my bedsit, was really starting to come up on this stupid pill, I wished warn others not to take.

I tried laying down on my bed, the drug had truly taken affect and I was now in full flight (tripping).

My head wanted to rest, (I was tired), head rushes were stacking on head rushes. The trip was taken me on a journey my body was rebelling against.

Taking hold was this trip, much like a group of friends want control over you if you let them, the not so good friends.

I was losing Arm & body sensations. Numbness in my arms & body areas, like I'd had a stroke. Making use of only the body left functioning. This was in every sense used of the word frightening.

I had no choice but to journey with 'her the trip'.

I opened my front door bedsit I stayed lived, walking 'downstairs' (I lived upstairs). I was 'coming up further' getting flashbacks, expanding head muscles, all sorts of scares.

Sure I'd experienced 'head rushes' with cannabis, (but head sways, head expansion swells, head swishing) swapped identity you exist as the (eyes) of Spiritless human! if born you wasn't!; so no 'Body' - you become the transit. This transit is in control of the body you intoxicated. The Air around us the Holy spirit. Chemical ways this transits Make-up; is the World or light years presence; (how looks); had not a human vessel you owned. The World existing as bare metal something us from a mortal existence; can not envisage on Earth. This was all. Very frightening on me.

I died already In my mind. Was alive in a body that was not grounded to the Simon connections I was familiar in safe journeys. And this did frighten me.

I kept walking out the front door. The trip was holding my hand in darkness 'found finding myself', still inside my room bedsit, trying to get a sleep then trying to go out, where more need I - get out go.

I was tired, really tired, my lateral self.

I am not saying all tripping experiences are of a bad Nature, just I was wrapped in cloaks of pure evil every time the real Simon wasn't fighting back, find sensation in toes fingers, giving myself Windmill arm Exercises, to bring Good Simon circulation, Grounded.

I was alone deepest 1st time my life in, I was scared real scared. This aloneness is not as frightening nevertheless; as an Autistic man's loneliness.

I couldn't phone no one cause I felt stupid. Warrior inside me, allowed me not to call out for help.

Like big brother airs you with, you can't call out find closeness happy. See family members, family others - bargaining excuses secured place.

I eventually remember leaving my bedsit. Hey this time I really had left the bedsit. I was Journeying.

I was scared. I was Simon. I can beat this I said.

I didn't want to die. I was losing the battle trip power on me. I'd not experienced power like this - it was excitement like of travelling fairgrounds roller coast rides trust in zero slides none.

I started to realize why good people turned into nasty people on my ((trip)). All the answers I was locking away. I had Questions too, piece of unfolded paper.

I could see clear middle eye, crystal clear answers, crisp answers. You'd not see had you been everyday you.

My hair upon leaving the Army had grown long curly thick, cause lots of hair, thick hair, big hair, runs in the Family.

I was drug stage of life in, so my hair was growing.

I was tripping bad my hair was coming alive, Joseph's amazing technicolour dream coat.

I see colours through hair locks mine moving slow mo, walking away out from Stamshaw. (Stamshaw area in Portsmouth I lived heading towards Tipner).

Morning arrives adversely Tripping badly just the same. My Motorbike (CB 125) unexplained is in an Alley way with me. I couldn't get out of this Alley. My heart was beating faster, walking forward walking back repeatedly panicking on a circuit. I knew I was there yet I experienced death.

My handle bars had ((Melted in front)) of me, kidding you not.

I was going forwards, then backwards in Alley way, continuous loop.

I was trying to back my Motorbike out of this Alley, I for no reason found myself in, but it wasn't having none of it. I was truly tripping.

I did get out the (VHS stuck rec.) - Alley eventually, I don't know how.

I was locked in a thought chamber, my own thoughts not releasing me go.

I did - gave up the fight trying to get out this Alley, cause I'm sure one of my thought's 'is/was' this is where you will die Simon.

I pretend see myself as Danny Glover (Captain Roger Murtaugh), movie Lethal Weapon.

He says time for you to die Roger, sitting his back to a tree, as Riggs (Martin Riggs) a supposed psycho nut job, chases the SAS man in the film Lethal Weapon.

4 movies were made.

I did let go in this alley, I wanted to die my way. If I'm going to die I want to die my way, (Capt Roger M) way - not yours, so I let go.

Had I of died, I was certainly still here, and found I was no longer in the Alley any or no more.

I was in-fact outside **Green Post pub** on **London Road.** (A Pub place, in Portsmouth).

I eventually rang my Mum, cause the Warrior within me had left, I didn't care about looking Stupid no more.

I just cared it was **((Over))**.

I just cared I was loved again, not fighting my battles lonely World as single man/boy no longer.

Soon surrounded by people who love me.

Magic Caps.

There was only one other drug I had taken a lot of, Magic Mushrooms. I smoked them, powdered them. In my tea, strained through a pair of lady's tights, soggy selections fresh.

As well as in tea making 'what was left' was dried out on the radiator and smoked.

Magic mushrooms are laced in LSD, so although considered a hippies delight, It can leave you (scarred powerless) if you're one of people that shouldn't mess with drugs. I did - I shouldn't. I gave up.

I'm not saying all drugs are bad, I'm not, cause a lot of people do have, 'quote' you know, (personality that works with the drugs).

I'm not openly gratifying, glorifying you thumbs up tickets. Drugs are weakness fighting a character you mould.

Just avoid drugs altogether if you don't want to lose your Character Identity stolen, cause that's what drugs did for me.

Sure I had a buzzing time but the real buzz, fires on all 4 corners of your Endorphins, the electroplated you, Natural in breathing.

Although completely enjoying softer drugs I was taken, I was getting forgetful, less caring towards others.

I lost all the principles Installed (into me) I took basic structure from the young age, didn't like the person I was becoming. Became.

Started when finished when.

I started as stated prior my drug use at 18.

Stopped aged 34/35 years of age.

I had abused my body the best part of 16 to 17yrs. I only then realised what a fool I had been.

I question myself why, why, why had I only stopped now, without giving in, clogged resin oil (baffling) my once sharp whistle.

Why?

Why only had I stopped when I'd satisfied myself 'I had done more than enough damage' to stump a Camel in its tracks, 1,000 Camel light years over, multiplied by a big number?

And why when I stopped was there not the rhythmic feel, of what good stopping point resembles? I was faith-ed out, fathoms below, only you kept those answers firing back.

My **Nanny Newell** always said to me when she was here alive: ('**Simon** you're **nobody's fool**'). And here, I am with the Joker Cards sat in ruining my deck.

I didn't like the person I was, I became, although only gave up the stinking Cannabis 6 to 8yrs ago, not exact timings. I've **not looked** back.

I just wish - I started not.

I started well in life. I was a role model student, fell at the fence, on a familiar slippery slope I am sure into becoming addicted to Cannabis. Said bluntly.

Not sure I know make wise 'when what people say', say: 'Cannabis is not addictive', not for them - their strong comes easily.

For me however, I had an addictive personality, craved the cannabis. Yet in Principle my Character should never of crossed Worlds. Temporary solutions I surrounded polished high, immersed in Water for the experience. I was split apart, trying to follow two very separate Journeys. 'In essence' I wanted to be both. In essence I wanted to be only one 'cause only one' is the source from the **good Fountain.**

I had a lot of fun times as well. It wasn't all bad, or

I'd not have enjoyed participating nasty habit which was helping me escape normal Society.

I don't want to talk about my drug side my life any more, it hurts me too talk about. I really do wish I could turn back the hands of time, the truth is I can't.

I just have to try and be the person I should have been 'had intentions be' (in start go), **from the early age.**

I'm not here to protest against drugs, nor do I care if you take drugs yourself.

I do care about people, **brought up** the **right way** though. If that sounds a bit contradict, then life is, especially mixed messages (we lost in - Autistic).

Led down the wrong paths a person takes drugs, should be only 'it wasn't influenced - on to him'.

He himself reached out for the drugs is when ok. Even then **not ok.**

I still don't like it. But see why you now must 'drug use' if indeed you are.

The drug user is more accepted experimenting, ((not involving another)), unless others are freely coming to him, should he run in circles at gigs e.t.c.

I feel so much better in life now (now ripped apart away from being in with the supposed in crowd), 'the ones I never felt a part of' for all the genuine I tried to then be.

I find freedom, open air, Sea walks, Camping, (uncontrolled activities) by strains what now you, 'don't have to' ((live up-to)). Simon's character is now chopped tree down.

I am really particularly against drugs, yet am no shining example, way I absconded abuse drugs. Should be, stays **shamed.**

I never quite knew just how much of myself ((I lost)) 'drug workings.' I am only now, after slow down 'of stop taking them', ((started to get memories seep back)) I lost - once apart of me.

In the once Natural mind state 'you'd find easy to' grab this 'Root Home', however a once easy Journey Natural mind ((I found hard)). For the wrong choices I kept taking, I now no longer am doing.

I am so thankful Jesus lives in my life now. Jesus is unrestricted, my drug on high enough. Gifts me white cloth loving. Pearls. 'Right' standing.

He alone is such an awesome God. He has forgiven me on sinful nature displayed over number of years, 17 to 18 years shown to be precise.

Pre-proposed expectations ((others set raised me so high)) 'they thought I'd be this person', **then I let them down.**

Asperger's roughly when?

So if I did have Asperger's at the young age 'and it wasn't diagnosed' you would thought might be recognised ((in my absences of Character)) through prolonged drug use, as one benefactor bringing out extra highlighted abnormalities.

I was so healthy when the younger man or boy, (without taking dreadful drugs) lived created own endorphins happiness joy.

I could have lived up-to 95 years old easily, (strength blanketed love I was brought up and gave).

Now my damaged body bad, will be lucky live 65. 62 is my best forecast as recovery comes slow.

Very possible being my own doctor, much earlier.

Taking drugs shortens your life by 20 to 25yrs 'unless environment' around your person, gives less or more back. Not joking you, that is my own fair kind assumption on humbled free.

Both my parents once smoke normal cigarettes, smoked over 40yrs. My dad only gave up when he had miniature inside unexplained heart attack, hospital weakly moves, with some nut job opposite him calling out to his wife.

You could not realistically find away ask my Dad stop smoking. The best approach, strange as may sound, was treat it as a good thing he did (not over complicate), something apart of Social fabric he is/was soft nature cares. My dad is easy going gentle, smoking was apart of this language we fit In, having a cigarette bonds. Sharing communing the 'laugh along easy approaches' we all care try be.

Loving your father as much as I do, you just accept they show love (by this sort of companionship smoking), smoking kinds, bond huddled flocks nestle.

I'd of preferred people who I do care about, (hadn't smoked). Given up thankfully presently.

My mother gave up smoking. My step dad, Paul, just before New Year came in 2014.

I personally think feel, 40 years smoking is time check say stop this now, the body does still repair itself, doctors shall disagree with me, I have to insist they are wrong.

(Reasons of care/love, I stay right).

40yrs of smoking, then stopping halt - might be your correct ingredient, that balances long longer life.

Nothing makes sense. We are told of certain amounts nicotine in our body (once or still), in medical journals, 'is required good, can help'.

I say cause I care about people, not cause I'm right. **I'm** choosing too be **right.**

Belief is mine. No matter what damage you have done as one individual to your body, (we may overcome put right), and so God sees trying you.

Giving you long age same you would have had (had not you of hurt damaged body yours)), scarred tissue hard repair. Not impossible.

Turning with God's white robes the last hope.

Ask baptism in water, from dirty tobacco yellow fingers.

Takes a lot of praying.

Springing governance 'being the caring' (late) though better late than never. Blank packets one message.

Yes oh Sovereign Lord, you are master the ((I am)).

Heal me Father, 'let me feel you around me' as I did in the square one moment, beginning of my life.

When you breathed your breath into my nostrils, gave me life. (Let me serve you Father), for the rest of my life, (not fall short), your Glory Sovereign King, of Kings.

Amen, Shalom.

You gave me a Gift of Life. Let no Sin rotten eggs Interrupt. Amen.

Reach out to me Father, so I may grab you with an 'outstretched arm'. Show me, teach me to Fish again Father, fill me with light not Idols you gave me from birth.

Never let me lose my shining glow, **'it took you along time, in entering a gifted shine, through my heart, "from you," the source of all sources'.**

Life not break me any more, oh Father when I am with you. Amen.

Private Newell.

Private Newell, 24881267, Sir. That was my army number I was enlisted as on enrolment into ((Intake 5)).

Private Newell get your head down - (no not sleep), that meant monkey crawl a safer position, leopard crawl prone position son - minimal exposure take cover, you're having Grenades thrown at you - shouting your buddies a warning ((Grenade)).

Thunderflashes also, blow this thing up, an only way people (really took stock listened), put under pressure, an army unit works together well.

It is when you see theory work (from classroom), to practical improvised situation come alive.

I loved army life (cause like) after each (Weekend), (drill night on a Thursday), where at an end of night or weekend!

Your Platoon comrades would swap stories, thoughts on ((way the weekend had gone)) 'or not gone so well', lesson's learned, drawn on.

On good numbers weekends away - not all, we would go up against other Hampshire-based - surrounding County ((Companies)) in Regiments for example. Our unit would think nothing of loading up 4x4 Lorry (HGV).

Setting out to Reading Barracks, to visit D Company for instance.

In history of ((our: Division - Brigades - Regiments - Battalions - Companies - Platoons - Squads)) - Names titled.

Army's belonging, buildings, Divisions, you came from served under. Names unwieldy staggered unnatural, movement forever changes.

In that history itself, can reveal quite the messy picture.

A.S myself I hate any form of Change, so do some Normals. Don't mean they're A.S. means they are, yes sensitive to (Change) - (siding A.S symptoms) shall be shown indiscriminate.

I was the Gunner of 3 Platoon, this meant if we were ambushed, Gunner had 75% fire power, over his comrades (with the S.L.R.'s at the time, that were in circulation). (S.L.R. is a - **self. loading. rifle**).

Although the boys called them (Silly.Long.Rifles).

The Regular army on some weekends away, would converge into a TA Unit such as ours sometimes, as would some veteran soldiers, who had army in the blood, would not retire.

They would not hang up their army boots, double knot just yet, because we knew these guys had least 25 to 35 years 'in our older boys of yet.'

The Regular Army was harder on a TA Unit, we would get called ((STABS)).

This stands for ((Stupid. Territorial. Army. Bastard.)) It was a little harsh, but hey ho, we were underdogs to them, right?

When you know they were doing the real thing, the Regulars were, they had real bullets fired at them, mostly 7.62mm Rounds.

So being called a ((STAB)), was worth the freedom of staying Weekend Warrior, we brushed off the things people say.

We just pushed our little chests 'out further', found the man in us, that told us we are still men.

Some TA Soldiers, were joining Regular outposts, with the (Regulars) on real exercises. So where you draw a line in calling people names matters no more.

My job was (the Gunner). I carried the heaviest weapon in Platoon, though not Carl Gustav 84mm (Anti-Tank weapon) heavy beast - perhaps why I suffer with **back problems** to this day.

The Gun, or more technically is 'Machine Gun' called a.k.a ((**GPMG**)).

That's ((General. Purpose. Machine. Gun)) to you and I. (Weight in excess of 30.5Ibs or 13.85KG, with a 50 Round belt).

The GPMG is a 51mm belt fed Gun, uses 7.62mm Calibre bullet round. The Weapon's 'uses' were (Light Weapon) or in 'SF Role' - that's (Sustained Fire).

The SF Role, meant the (Gun) was Mounted on a Tripod I believe, typically firing 'Tracer Rounds' Red fiery glow, very bright - ((fired every 5th round)) helps Aiming, especially come Night time. Mounted on vehicles moving Land Rover perhaps.

The Command (Watch my Tracer) was common language I was accustomed to hearing bellowed by a (Sniper) in the wings - as we watch lay down fire our target made known.

The GPMG, when under attack was manned as a 2 man team, me the Gunner, my buddy to my Right, feeding Belts of usually 100/200 Rounds, tied from 'shoulder to hip', like in the Rambo movies when not in use.

You see Stallone, Kris crossed ammo, hanging from his body parts.

The ((**NO 2 man**)) 'to my GPMG' job, was clearing any blockages, making sure flow of the Rounds in long belts were entering the guns housing 'flat' for example.

He may well be responsible cleaning my Weapon, lubrication was Important 'so Oiling another job his doing.'

Also if I'm getting tired, (my No 2 man) can take over 'I do the Job then as No 2", we are trained in both, alternative thinkers.

Should the GPMG, find itself used in an SF mode ((Mounted on Tripod)). The GPMG with a two-man crew lays down 750 Rounds 'per minute' at ranges 800m (light role), up to 1800 metres (SF role).

That's lots of range for any ones dollar believe me.

The GPMG can be carried by foot soldiers, employed as a Light Machine Gun (LMG), trust me it's anything but.

You carry this sucker, through dust & dirt, marshlands, swamps, bogs, wet terrain - sinks you a foot passed soles of your feet. You know the true meaning of pain, carrying our ((G.P.M.G)).

It's all very well talking about the pains we go through, the carrying of equipment in the army as one point to make, whilst downing your 2nd or 3rd Pint of **beer**, to someone who never has carried heavy loads, 'just laughed off in chatter'. Whilst the real men contain the pain, and so laugh along with you.

Not only this whilst out on patrol, high risk areas 'you

carry her, not just from the Hip' you are carrying her, (The GPMG) from butt into Highest part of Right Shoulder tucked hard in.

A Real Recoil kickback she has, it can break a man's shoulder, ((highly Elevated your Gun must be)), be that S.L.R or G.P.M.G.

Entering built up areas 'requiring the ears to listen, faintest smallest of sounds', a twig snapping, a stone falling, 'looking through your (**sites**) at all times', beads of sweat.

Not resting your machine gun, keeping your elbows high, 'it is pain' this is training a Soldier one instance (I've shared) goes through. Making good use of eye contact, hand flagging trusted soldiers of friendship find easy bonds.

It's all too easy 'not give a Soldier' proper respect he deserves, when person normal civilians sit sitting in comfortable armchairs, eating 200g bag Tortillas with Hot Salsa Dips. Brought down ALDI's or LIDL's.

Left hand munching, 'right hand Gaming' on Play-Station - X box.

I had a 14" to 18" long Machete strapped to my Bergen for clearing hard built up areas undergrowth, springy twisted sun snapped trees, no further apart than I can open both arms away from my body.

The Machete was a handy bit of kit, I bought mine in Scotland, whilst in Edinburgh, one weekend. We were given **R&R** days, that's, Rest & Recuperation.

This was a day/days given, whilst on an Annual Camp each year.

Or it was simply on Weekends away say 1/2 Days - with given R&R days hours built in to suit the fabricated weekends.

Such an R&R ((was merited earned by hard work)), our comrades had sweated. This was a time where a Soldier could stop playing Soldier, and relax.

My two closest friends in 3 Platoon were Mark Ray - Steve West Thomas. I was 17-yrs-old, they were 28 and 32-yrs-old.

Each others' (backs) covered - we had, some more than others. Steve trained with me outside of Army hours, we run together every other night, 3 mile runs.

Special nights aside set in pushing 12 Mile runs, circuits we chose on night, was random always. This was done at times carrying substantially heavy Bergen (Rucksacks).

Sergeant Barwis.

I loved Sgt Barwis. Was our Sergeant - P.T. Instructor combined, originally he was from Regular Army, before came back Civilian life - working as a telephone engineer.

Now part time Army - normal Weekend Warrior role - 3 Stripes proudly sewn his arm.

He was what Sergeant resembles - in my book. If Sergeant was said to 'have a certain look' people were looking for, his what you'd picture in mind - (a sergeant stands up).

Good-humoured, hard when wanted, real glowing in army life. When he ran 'his feet glided', not touching ground, had known as spring in his step.

I see this man turn from nice Sgt Barwis ((Steve loved by many)), to giving someone a right dressing down, 'a bollocking' at snap fingers. It was enough to put fear of God in me/you.

I was always looking to make 'The Good Soldier', I as one reason tagging.

I gave no one an excuse to dress me down. I kept my head down, got on with the job. One, cause I didn't want hassle, 2, because hey, I was this person anyway, naturally happy energetic.

Yet described as Normal in TA life, I stood out as - different. I was noted from regular Normal.

French Foreign Legionnaire.

Sergeant Jones, or 'Ging' to his higher friends (French Foreign Legion), asked me receive a Trophy '3 Platoon had Won', (might have been A Company) whole 1, 2, 3 Platoons family unit Battalion - or as a Regiment - my mind forgets - won together).

We were standing on Parade 'at ease, stand easy', soldier mode.

Than as the afternoon proceeded. Highly decorated ranks came too unfold: Generals - Brigadiers - Captains - Lieutenant's - Officers were moving in - rosewood feel baton Canes, pace swagger, sticks under arm, men of brass filling (square) and Presentations Awards began.

Platoon - Platoon, 'Shun ... This was crying out, calling bellow scream to gather troops ranging low/ high pitch squeals, that happened to raise a few comical eyebrow laughs, usually from Sergeant Major echoing. Wearing very distinguished, leather 2" wrist band shows Kings Crown, (from as close as I observed).

Colour Sergeants - wore Colourful 2" wide trouser belts, looked military Aesthetic.

Down to Sergeants, Corporals, Lances, all had powers, pulling in-line a Platoon. Platoon, 'Shun. 'Company/ Platoon'. Attention eyes front.

Talking Colour Sergeants I forgot mention my confidant ((Colour Sergeant Wing)), this man I held respect, see family man, brother, imagery facial feature (brothers look like this).

I would always go to my Colour Sergeant should problems do arise.

He was the man sort them out, have his Secretary draft papers. A Father Figure if you will to all 3 Platoons in A Company. A man powering good your way.

'As was our Sergeant Major. Dad.'

So from 'Platoon' to "Platoon, 'Shun" was a movement from open legs ((to Platoon Shun)) 'where both legs were in together - not legs apart.'

I walked forward gave an illusive awaited nod - like Princess Leia smiled at me, Medals ceremony end of Star Wars. (Han Solo - Luke Skywalker - feel).

Gave my Generals & Lieutenants the hardest of Impressive Salutes, you ever did see.

It was sharp clean crisp Salute never forgotten this day, in always present. (Stays abreast with me.)

Ginger Jones was so Impressed with me, he took me to one side, personally gave me gratification, this built me as a Soldier. Encouragement I needed.

The respect where respect's due Ging wanted me to know.

Handed out 'respect', 'where respect's are due', not Lightly freely given, you had to earn those make you feel goods.

So I was in a band of men now growing in strength, Showing who Simon was, (showing me I am equal to my brothers in arms), no matter of rank, unarmed I am Special. You are Special.

Simon was growing in 'my Comrades & Ging.'

'Strength in them is now in me.'

I am Proud with confidence, because the Army made, a person I am agreeable.

What stage did you say you had Asperger's again?

If at this stage in my life I was told I had Asperger's, than little was I told or aware.

Had you of mentioned the word Asperger's, I'd have said what's that, 'is that a pizza topping or something?'

It was only in ((Mill House Hostel)), I was to find out what Asperger's meant.

And so my learning in Asperger Way's began, when I was more mentally aware of my Actions told, and why only now I could understand why firstly I myself, was so different to others.

I think had I not been in a ((Hostel)), seen the Doctor, it is possible I would 'never' have been diagnosed with Asperger's. I'd have been described a weird Normal instead.

People would know, I'm somewhat different to Neuro-typical 'but a diagnosis' ((could have gone unrecognised)).

You will find in this World today, if you ask any Doctor, or Aspergeric people in Chat room Communities on computer, they would agree with me Is my gut feel (a **lot** of **cases** do go **unrecognised**).

I was one of the Lucky ones who stumbled on my Diagnosis, in pure chance.

I would encourage you, should you know someone, a friend, or Related people, showing mannerisms you may read up on, see an article in a Magazine about, you steer them into making an appointment. With the right connections.

Then people can stop labelling him/her weird. Cause now they will know why they are Weird, tread hopefully careful-er around.

The words we express are best written in a book, than spoken tongue, which had me motivated reason I seek-ed out an express tool.

The value of words given in a book, the expense it incurs, time takes crafting your book, is listened too more so 'as it's not Sofa talk'.

It's a road map in collective thoughts, you can't wash away it's solitude solid, the only second best high is recorded coverage of your words like MP s for example in House of Commons, watched like hawks a talking book read as they perform - said quicker messages without Chapters - published just by standing there opening ones cake hole.

I often ask myself how much conviction, passion in

MP's speeches on behalf their constituents information prepared when the cameras switched off (do they, would they) freely give away ((to help the same - in first parallel)). Not only when supported by 'Red Rec light is On' when applause jaw dropping, ((here here)) - is gaining them voices of charm suited dickie bows. I came back to only one conclusion of old - (Information isn't free), yet it should be free - is quickest way tasks/ jobs turn around complete - yet no cigar does the MP win, had his message shared (uncopyrighted). Leave all glory to him on your way out - this time unfortunately not.

It sure takes less time (speaking your Book) rather than (Writing your Book) - yet only when you're lime lighted a recording of sort Interview backed evidence feathering ones own nest... that a book gives back the same - with extra physical presence - reward you can't collect at the ATM had you loosely gave all your words away for Zero members of public.

Writing book expressed normally over a 2 year period, showing you as Simon in 2-year spans. The start and finish efforts is money well spent. I heard someone say once it's so expensive publishing a book. I thought this nonsense - had I said all I communicate over to you 'my reader', (open language - lips freely flapping) then how would you know value words collective as you remain stronger than Oak Tree, stay bearing (seen evergreen), not disappearing leaves. A book that's not there.

Also a Book gives you more chance to altar, make changes to mistakes, that you can't have a second chance for (in Sofa talk) or down the shops giving away your feelings free.

(Sofa talk, explain: a bunch of people you entrust 'call friends' you unburden yourself on).

A book will/gives you, the Author, a chance altar make changes, speaking voice running holy spirit throughout, the higher you.

Unblock keep untangled, a narrow gorge light in answers - is this channel, or something else.

'Whereas words on Sofa laughing cackling out' are not show-boated harmony channels. As you less time channelling developing your answers.

This is what it takes, bring you a not immediate answer, in shining as the immediate answer you thought was right with now added extra polish.

Otherwise you're asking a posed Question to be addressed more quickly downloaded answered than a fast Internet (s) provider (IP).

Communication can not supply on demand like this, sure I can give you quick instinctive accuracy - if you're looking for something more Quick, immediate, finer answers pleasing your - Ears, Tuning Forks, cause I took no pause before response.

Only technology moves on, not the human mind now turning. Quick answers are respected more so.

An Oven cooking half a bag of Potato Wedges won't taste right, hurrying along the cooking process, by firing her up to Gas 9. The quickened answers.

You leave at recommended Gas mark.

Wisely you lay wait, like a Gurkha scrim netted for your tasty Wedges baked to satisfaction. You wait for answers to develop, not cook your answers hurried along, on Gas mark 9.

Mill House hostel for the homeless.

Mill House 'where I was Diagnosed', was a sort of halfway house for the homeless, and prison reform, reform a prisoner back into Society.

They really looked after you 'Mill house'. I later moved onto other hostels part of the same organization.

(Two Saints) was the organization I believe.

There was a 2nd hostel - Foster Rd Hostel.

And a 3rd Hostel I moved into was Locksway Rd Hostel.

Mill House was seen as rougher, all mixes, warps of

live entered. Then you were moved on to ((Foster Road Hostel)), after about a year or two, it was different for all.

Foster Road was a step-up from the previous, to those who proved their worth. In the stages we were all developing in Mill House.

Mill House reminded me bit of Oliver Twist. Where we were all just made to get on. The food was amazing, out of this World, **4 square Meals a day** were always set out.

'Breakfast, Lunch, Main Dinner', with a kind of 'snack feast' later on through the Evening.

I enjoyed my time, in Mill House, it taught me a lot, in how I was developing. We freely walked around like we owned the place - of course we didn't. The Mill House Staff took care of Authority, a Discipline which maintained.

There were I think, 2 Pool rooms, 2 to 3 TV Rooms, where you could freely walk around, mix & mingle with others, get in with - the wrong sorts, if you were not careful. Though I will say the (Wrong sorts) were good people - just be yourself works.

Asperger's revealed itself to me in a slow hand, turning later on 'a year later in' in the **(Mill)**. Timings are shadowed. Therefore by no means accurate. Though yes, (a year or so) **before diagnosed** in the **(Mill)**.

I would mostly keep myself to myself. I learnt from the older boys, who would you see not converge out his territory. Yes, a mix of people may be with him.

But the crowds dispersed, & reformed at unknown times. You knew when the big dogs/tiny dogs were around, druggies, timid folk, big boys, soft lads, decent persons, fashionables, Jokers, the ever so quiets, the concentrated, the gambler, the respecting kinds, the farting, fitness types, there was no ending this list, all sat in one TV Room - or Out and About around the (Mill). People from places:

Scotland.. Northampton.. London.. Hull.. Ireland..

Oxford.. Isle of Wight.. Portsmouth.. Leeds.. Bristol...

Manchester.. Wales.. Devon.. Liverpool.. Southampton.. Chi - Chichester.. Winchester.. You'd not end this list.

People come together at our Hostel as One. (Accents) a list not ending.

It was during the quieter times I would sit with the older boys.

They'd do Crosswords, watch Countdown on TV, taking pen & paper into TV rooms, in aiding solving the Conundrums. Richard Whiteley/Carol Vorderman ((then hosted)), back in the day. Around 1997 - 2003, not exact dates here rough guideline my time in the (Mill).

The other hostel, Foster Road was a 2nd stage hostel move on.

Locksway Road hostel - final 3rd stage hostel.

You had to go through each stage properly, before you were given the power to move on. Eventually the idea is, if you kept your nose clean, you hopefully can eventually 'move on, into your own flat'.

Given the Key training, in how able to look after yourself. The Development programmes you processed through, to reach the Happy Doors.

I was over the moon in 2003 when I had a few Interviews, later receiving a few letters, saying I can move into my ((new Studio flat)) I had been allocated, by Portsmouth City Council.

My new flat was in (Portsea) Southsea, Portsmouth. Ground floor flat.

Opening - 'my front door', my 1st experience in life, of owning my own little flat.

It felt amazing, surreal, it really did. Though I never show others I'm excited, in-case the very often jealousy seen - says hello.

Opening (my flat door), or washing the dishes in my new

kitchen. I had a great view sighted outside my patio of Spinnaker Tower located at Gunwharf Quays.

Frostbite.

On a Weekend away one weekend through the year, back between 1989 - 1991, the dates a little muffled, 'must been Winter time', I know this as it was bloody freezing. We had driven down from Portsmouth, driven up, in-fact debused from our 4 x 4's. (Debused 'army term used' means! 'dismount').

Then - Fell in, process all Platoon's line up, smarted up by shuffling their feet, so spacing's in-between each soldier smartened up.

((By extension of left arm from side out, elevated to shoulder level soldiers in row, helped find your spacing)).

(Tips of fingers should be just touching your colleagues shoulders within reason. 'If not', you required another reshuffle of feet or till alignment runs).

You're looking basically troops lined on your sides in your row. In front rows, behind rows - squaring symmetrical so even looked diagonals, run straight.

Till whole of 3 Platoon were in presented enough way, that the Officer in question who is giving debriefings, ((the run down, or overview info given)). Our Platoon, was considered neat & tidy, talk to his 'one group body of men', women, as One whole Uniform.

((He shadow chisels a picture)) 'in each soldiers mind', that we universally had some understanding how the weekend is been graphed out. By planners, Officers, commands trickling down by the higher Heads reaching us. Weeks, months in the plans advanced previous graphed shape around.

Leading up to where we were, now standing in line.

Platoon. Platoon, 'shun, shouted out a senior in command, a bellow from the pit of his stomach.

The ((brigadier)) Sergeant Major or Lieutenant, 'comes on

Parade' salutes the brigadier, (or high ranking official) as either one of these commanders now, walks off.

Leaving 'one commander,' to talk as a whole to 3 Platoon. On that matter, this would include 1 Platoon plus 2 Platoon e.t.c.

'Stand at ease. Stand easy,' the lieutenant now hollows, (ringing in, resounding in each), all our ear lugs.

At this stage we have all had a good breakfast an hour before, from the canteen barracks, usually sausages, eggs, beans, bread/butter, hash browns, bacon, scrambled eggs, toast, tomatoes. Were all items on a typical menu, in the mess halls.

You line-up choosing accordingly, usually this will be self service, other times, you are served by the unit cooks in charge. It was the one meal that set all soldiers on their feet for the day, before their stomachs were grumbling again, at 12:00pm midday to 1pm.

The time in our 'talking down debriefings', is now roughly going on at ((06:15hrs)) standing at ease.

We woke at times around 04:45hrs - 05:30hrs depending. We had been up all of 45mins ((was fed)), while now our lieutenant was debriefing us.

Debriefings would usually last 5 to 10mins sometimes much longer. We were on an '**Escape & Evasion weekend**' on Salisbury Plain, Wiltshire. It was bloody freezing.

Even with my northern Ireland gloves on, I was frosty jacks, trembling from lips, knee, legs.

We'd had our debriefing spelled out to us now, were quickly fell out. (Dismissed turn to right, by way of a pivoting of ones feet, again quickly marched off). **Left, left - left .. right .. left ..** 'were our timings.'

This was all going on at a time **before** I was **diagnosed** with - the beautiful **Asperger's** I delight in, before I was informed Simon has Asperger's.

No one in my Regiment see my Asperger Colours, living with them - in me.

I was still a young boy. The Asperger's in me, if you will, hadn't turned tumorous yet.

It was as I explain it (in dormant state), it was not triggered off yet.

I am sure my drug taking triggered 15-20% portion of it in me, or at least added, to an already conditioned mind misdiagnosed, cause no diagnosis was logged, to be found in me later.

My drug taking days never lapsed into my Army days, they were very separate tea cakes.

So this led me believe, as normal boy with the right love, my parents - the army gave me, and they did.

Whilst I was growing up into, turning out into a real nice young man, spoken properly, a little shy, reserved.

I knew no better. I was not a leader, I would have been your follower, led easily.

Led me believing (A.S is a condition) 'actively seen' when conditioning subjected is not conditioning his.

On saying: my condition worked in my favour sporadic. I was probably without blowing my own trumpet, one of fittest young men in our outfit, follower or leader.

I had respect for my elders.

I had a built in intelligence as a boy. It didn't however show as intelligence till I was Aspergic aware, then found ((my confidence **grew**)), now I had a '**diagnosed explanation**' that wouldn't drag down an (unconfident intelligence) I let sag before.

My new diagnosis gave me new meaning to my life. I was confident enough now ((to show intelligence)), cause I wouldn't be broken by others ever again, now that I was given (my own mind tools). I solved better with aspergic love allowed to blossom, my better working methods was partly due to working with my ((Aspergic mind tools I had)), not my Normal mind tools I tried saying I hadn't.

Flopping failing in Normal mind set, 'I bagged my Normal

mind tools away', discontinuing their use.

Had I shown, ((lights of intelligence)) in what I once considered was my normal self, then it didn't run in parallel to what others appreciated.

You see I was ((un - confident as normal Simon)), cause I was trying to be intelligent, in normal circles, that went against my own natural grain.

My intelligence as a boy if it was there ((wasn't showing)) un-confident hid behind tree.

For any response I'd be almost denied, had I shown a healthy tree, was why perhaps I never grew confidently Normal, confidently intelligent.

It was showing as 'fitness only', an enthusiasm I shared in army life my intelligence was.

By this I mean my outstanding asset in the Army was my capability/strength, ripping out of me. I was real in Rhythm with life, encouraged routines I fly through, (Why? Cause was once allotted me), so I gave flying colours.

Routines were not a problem then, especially with a boyish love I thought others loved me for, made routines easy to Sail.

Routines then not a problem now I have Asperger's. Though the routine powers I excelled at once, left me more as time passed me by, loved (same ways) sidelined me. So did routines, unless I worked personal Interest I bore my barrel.

So more my Asperger's was taking a grip, especially in guitar playing days (I literally fought to learn) cause government problems 'spokes' distracting my keen learning mind, not running concurrent fastenings a mind they pulled in line.

Asperger's was taking hold faster ((controlled)) - whilst only **compulsive obsessive** behaviorism routines in Guitar **remained.**

'Ordinary normal routines left me'.

Especially with lesser love. Conforming not allowed Special Simon, which I thought was normal. But to fit in the ordinary World, you all, apparently must look the same. Given no Special treatment - only heightens my Asperger's I have no doubt.

Hindering an already Asperger's softer than most guys.

I was to be left powerless, lost a part of my brain that once seemed like second nature.

Yes routine hadn't completely left me, guitar is a system of routines.

We play songs in exercises playing 5 note, 7 note scales in all routines.

As are: Finger exercises, Chord progressions, 12 bar cycles, your bag of licks & riffs, you personally selected into your armoury all based loosely around our ((**Brother Routine**)).

I hear you calling out to me, so Simon what I don't understand about your Asperger's is: how could you not of known 'you yourself' in your own right - not know you had - something wrong with you?

If we are saying Asperger's is now the considered wrongful state of mind, looked down the nose from Society's high hills.

Well to give you an answer, your ears pleased, that you feel release of energy leaving you. Ears clearing canal a sighing relief, I answer you in this way.

May answer you in another way, should you ask me weeks later, here's your answer for today only, please take it be satisfied.

My Answer then.

Look I have never had a dividing line in life. Where on this side of a River Severn. River Thames e.t.c, I was Normal Simon 100%.

Then (the Army roping me in), sailed my kit over to other side River (in black bin liners) kept water proof.

Breathe... and this side of the rivers edge. I was 100% Aspergeric after a Diagnosis. ((Mill House Hostel, where my Diagnosis was made aware)).

You see I was Aspergic before diagnosis it must be assumed, though it took years before someone recognised - my A.S.

Having a diagnosis called: ((Mild Asperger's)). Tells you my Asperger's (**was Mild**), harder assumed it is to spot.

I very nearly never went to Mill House, it was only on a whim from a Bed & Breakfast I moved out of. Cause I had incurred some debt with my landlady.

Basically **I hopped it...**

Turning up at the gates of Mill House one night. I remember it well it was pissing down cats & dogs. I felt like Oliver twist please Sir. Do you have a spare room?

No. Come back when the Wizard is a Wizard who will serve, was a felt answer 'through the hatch, from a member of Mill House Staff'.

So I walked around St Mary's Road all night 'collar turned up', scarf padded out criss-crossed, keep chest warm.

((St Mary's Rd. A Central well-known Road in Portsmouth.))

The next day arrived I was literally at Mill House, banging on their Iron door knocker, just as soon as Mill House wakened.

I filled in a form, given a refreshing cup tea. Interviewed, shown my room, 'that was to be start of my Mill House life encounter'.

'Had I hadn't of hopped it' from the landlady, **I'd not** of had **my diagnosis.** Reiterated.

So to say I was normal this side of the (fence), as explained. Then after diagnosis, on other side of this damn fence, snap of fingers I was now an Aspergic - is simply not true.

I became Aspergic aware - a leading up that declined my Normal ways. Gradual process Shedding my skin like a snake would.

I will always have a Normal and Aspergic life element, revving through. As for one: I am diagnosed Mild Aspergic Sufferer.

2: the older I get, getting... the more shedding of the normal skin, is not staying with me. It's a water bucket filling, becoming heavier in Asperger's, older & older I become became.

Meanwhile back on **Salisbury Plain**, I was freezing my nuts off. We had just been dismissed by the Company's Lieutenant.

Pictures left with us, to how Officers above us, told us our Weekend would pan-out.

It was Saturday, we had undergone a hive of activities, before the time was now (1pm) to anything up to 3pm.

Assault courses, shooting practice, not necessarily in this order, from mind memory, were typical things going on over a weekend away with the T.A.s.

We were now in buzzed mood, playing out the **Escape** & **Evasion Weekend** we solely were there for, ((a weekend declared as more Special, non like others, of basic assault/shooting courses, basic what to expects, still yet spontaneity)).

We were led by, **Private Mark Ray** who could have easily been a Corporal from as much as my memory tells me, **he had** completed his **2 week NCO Cadre**, and was now leading the boys. Ever watched as his leadership was shaping, the new man he broke into.

We were approaching many derelict buildings, bombed out buildings that looked like they had seen a few thousand Soldiers come & go, expansion of the years.

We walk gingerly through the undergrowth, uneven ground, a silent code, is maintained, ((hand signals & a good eye contact maintained)), our rifles are cocked, ready for action.

My sights are up, my hands are still bloody freezing, my rifle is moving from left to right, in a moving arch. Where my rifle points, my eyes follow in a left to right... **bang bang ban.** Get to cover, Mark our Corporal shouts. We get our heads down, we have taken the low ground in a prone or half knelt position, depending on the soldiers view.

Thunderflashes are hurled nailing us down, the Air is filling with red pinkish smoke, ((smokers, to help us or the enemy advance)).

I reach for a Grenade in a pouch attached to my Webbing. My hand **could not** pick up the **Grenade**, it was in the **1st stages** of **Frostbite.**

I touched one hand to feel the other, both were numb blocks of ice, welded cold.

Double the strength cold, Birds Eye Fish Fingers reach. My hand was like a potato that was left at the back of freezer, double hard, frozen solid. My potato hand had double below zero sensation. It was dangerously cold, I kidding you not.

I'm sure this is why I have problems to this day with my hands, the numbing sensations I incur periodically, now in the latter life. Twinges, here and there irregular uncomfortable sometimes sharp quick pains.

All triggered from Frostbite. This was not diagnosed as so, but I know what Frostbite is, I was you might say 'too proud stubborn, too young' in telling.

The hand of mine, was not picking this cold lumpy weighted Grenade up, searching around my pouch no sensation below half my arm nearest my hand. Hand muscles sleeping, locked closed weighted potato. My right hand inactive, no one solitary movement.

I had arm movement, I had leg movement, both hands were inactive. My rifle was held merely with the weakening strength of my inner wrists, pressing into below chill factor 'rifle'.

A crust of Ice tissue, was formed around the Rifle's Butt shiny cold metal parts. This did not deter us, we were Soldiers. My gloves heavy useless.

I was at every opportunity, I wasn't shot at. 7.62mm Rounds, whistling past my Kevlar (helmet).

'Warming in increments' ((when could)), rubbing of the hands, blowing hot breath in.

I carried on advancing using (cover and go) buddy buddy system, closer to the Enemy. Reaching we were, buildings firing up barb-wired stairs. The Enemy enshrouded a defence between us & them.

Mark is hit by lobbing **Thunderflash**, ringing stunted my ears. Mark was blinded by brightness a Thunderflash leaves, brighter than Welder not wearing his mask. Mark was down, I had gone temp deaf.

I proceeded to fire 7.62s up the stair-wells. Retreat, return fire, retreat, return, whilst rest of lads in our Platoon bundled. Were now closing In, taking off their Jackets, throwing them over hard, en-laced Barbed Wire, the Enemy resided themselves.

They had advantages of high ground shooting down. Shooting up put us at - disadvantage, the courage we showed gave us advantage.

We were soon throwing smokers. Over throwing the Enemy, Flushing them out, taken prisoners to the not fallen cable tying enemy wrists, finding maps they had in possession, information...any small clues, radio ops, extra ammunition we would lay our hands on, Pyrotechnics available.

Marching off sorry arsed Enemy.

The whistle was blown at it felt 4pmish, declaring end ex.

(End of Exercise, meant **mission complete**).

The enemy were lightly tortured, though the Geneva Convention, tells us to treat all prisoners with respect.

So a Soldier is not in court, explaining his torturous ways. All people should be treated fairly, as should Aspergic people.

The Geneva Convention, was created to look after soldiers taken prisoner of War.

The Geneva Convention is meant to guarantee a prisoner's status.

I do say meant.

Rifle Tranquillity.

Cleaning my Rifle in the field was tranquil, it's a time where all the boys in your Platoon, or as One whole Battalion, Regiment e.t.c, would feel the free open fields.

The wind whistling through, 'blowing the grass blades', an untold directions.

The morning smell of fresh Dew on the grass. In Winter, the frozen stiff bunched grass, the white sheen of frost.

Summer was best. Winter's best for other varying reasons, 'though were cold on one's butt'. Although the boys ((had knee pads)), should they choose this luxury, (pads bought from a sports shop usually).

It had the affect of effectively helping not get your combats wet, stones stuck in knee caps, kneeling uneven broken grounds, yet clumsy in walking running, sang a downside should you be pinned down under attack, or not much time to release pack away the 'Pads'.

Unless come employed quick release ((Velcro)), a favourite option for many things military.

Best grass time of day cleaning one's Rifle, was just in reach of the morning time, fresh Dew on the grass, on a field that was covered in empty 7.62mm bullet rounds.

Just the smell of empty, Live or blank Rounds ((bullets)) was what gave the Army 'as one instance', the smells you associate with Army life. What 'made had' you coming back for more, and or the uniforms had a distinct Army smell to them, especially the Hairy Mary's. These were warm Army shirts working dress No 2s hairy itchy woollens, not cotton variety used more on Parade smart.

Target practice produced lot of these Empty Rounds seen on field, these fields were of Acres, Acres and Acres. The eye lost vision that the fields carried on,

on, On. The beautiful energy places I visited in my 2-year spell in T.A. 's made you stand up take notice, of what's in England's back garden, had you never ventured out, a radius of your home. The T.A. 's gave you many opportunities to travel with them, not only this, they cared to look after you.

Here we were plonked in the middle of a small area, 'spread out' cleaning Rifles when chances came. Camouflaged like Christmas trees through the long grass, crouching crawling all movements, including good communications advancing on Enemy positions.

If there was a threat!!!

We would have, ((Gunners in say 3 Corners)) of our Triangle within a Circle, whilst cleaning our Rifles in middle 'the protection we put out'.

Battle Ready at any time to stop what we were doing, re-assemble the guns /Rifles Working parts, back into main Rifles body, should an attack be immanent, battle-Fatigued or not, you got on with it.

We would have, as part of our Rifle cleaning Kit, ((Rifle Pull through s)) a long piece of rope a good metre long, specially made for rifle, inserting ((cleaning cloths)) used with a weight on one end.

'That weight,' drops into your rifle's long barrel, a snapped open S.L.R/G.P.M.G cleans Spiral, well-machined engineered inner long spout. This barrel is a non mechanism chamber. This was all done by minute or so of rapid ((pulling the rope back & fourth)) from entrance point, 'to point out'.

Used in both 'left & right hands' ((the pull-through)),

with 'cleaning cloth' in rope, cleaning rifle's Spiral. The Rhythms you cleaned too ((pressed held between)), one's knees, thighs.

Last process was dropping the one-sided weight rope, through rifle's Spiral in holes diameter where you've heard the expression, ((I had 20 bullet rounds in Magazine, one up the Spout)).

Rifle's (spiral spout) was cleaning entrance point, 'or at least in my language it were! how I might Interpret' pulling through our ropes. Rifles broken open, if you like. Last cleaning process was ((weighted pull through, dropped in spiral's hole)) 'one direction only' rapidly giving it 10 or so - one directional pull through' s, not back & fourth 1st process we encountered.

We then would find where 'most light shone' from around in the field, with a squinted eye, looked through Spiral's area ((satisfying myself see she was gleaming)), before declaring yourself. That's enough of that.

The Rifles/Machine Guns did need cleaning, mainly due to Carbon build up, after a long weekend away e.t.c. This was not always easily removed.

Such household items used clean our Rifles, for example 'Scotch Brite' was one best I found, (Brittle Green pads used in washing up dishes).

The (Gas Plugs) were the worst 'cleaning wise', caked on carbon.

Our Sergeant showed us a neat trick, (Ginger Jones from French Foreign Legion). He would buy small bottle of 'Tabasco sauce', this stuff was sent from Heaven, it actually ate away at carbon, a couple minutes with Scotch Brite combined, worked wonders.

It is amazing tricks trade you learn. From passed on tried proofed methods, from our Fore-father soldier friends. Although this along with Gel acidic other products on market, was a keep it under your hat trick not to be seen done by your passing Armourer Staff Sgt man in Armoury. Though most soldiers used some kind

(Carbon) removal products, as did I. It was, dare I say, a silent acceptable. As over time prolonged usage of Gel acidic, even (Tabasco sauce) quick magic solutions, eats pits away at gun's metal. 'Not much' to its side effects though, considered a no no.

Brass Monkeys.

Would get cold out on Weekends, especially cleaning cold Rifles, so lot of the boys wore finger-less black gloves. Not only did they keep you warm, they really did look the part.

We would most often have a 'Signal's operative' in field with us. A 'Medic', at least One in each Platoon was assigned with us ((bandages, 1st Aid kits)), worn Arm pocket most often, or a Tin of First Aid 'must haves' we'd carry on our person.

Or in our Webbing, quick access, though tendency with 1st Aid Kits, was they would rattle around hell of a lot, so cotton wool was another neat trick in padding out these tins, thus easy used in Medical Emergencies.

We all had 1st Aid Kits, though One Senior was at least Qualified assigned to us.

Calling in Mother Earth.

The Radio Operatives guy, could call in Air Strikes, get us moved the hell out of there, should we find ourselves ambushed for example.

And a: **H**otel. **E**cho. **Li**ma. **I**ndia.

Charlie. **O**scar. **P**apa. **T**ango. **E**cho. **R**omeo.

Was called to our hideout, smoke signals, flares used, helicopter sights on, see us.

Problem with becoming Signal Operatives in your Unit Platoon Is, he is 1st person Snipers exampling target, in taking out.

This remains true about Gunners, my Job. 75% your Platoons fire power comes through this guy by your side.

When you think G.P.M.G. Fires off, Rates up to 750 rpm. Belt fed, that's again lot of Fire power.

The G.P.M.G could be fired from hip, or most noticeably seen used with Bipod, fixed part G.P.M.G.'s feature, used in Prone Position, (on your belly's position).

The Helicopters used in T.A. & REGS were, from what I remember:

The Chinooks, Wessex, Puma, Links.

We were in Perth Valley's of Scotland, helicopter riding through Mountainous low valleys after exercises had us radioing in on telephone. Then our bird, Majestic landed, shadowed bird of prey windy landing, loading my (SF GPMPs) I raced excitedly.

I remember thinking is this (heli bird) going to take off. It felt strange being inside a helicopter - I looked out my side window one time, surprised to find we'd left - were way up. Scotland never looked so beautiful as it did at this special moment, gripping my gun hard I looked around inside a metal-padded shell all over my eyes followed. On 2 week Cadre away, apart and parcel 2 week annual camp went away on in turn, helped us earn a ((**BOUNTY**)) once a year.

A Bounty was a given amount money to each Soldier, **In:** 1st. 2nd. 3rd years of substantial amounts.

You only achieved this Bounty, by completing tasks set out through the year attending **Annual camp**, would be one then.

Those higher in the chains of command loved the power 'they were giving' by knowingly you're in their Control for Whole 2 weeks. **Beast** you, they surely may. Though stress wasn't bullied beasting. 'Necessary' beasting brung out "**the you**" they wanted to see. So a degree must exist so you stay a Good Soldier and I was always best behaving.

This is how forming/breaking bonds pushed to our best Circulated.

Map Reading.. N.B.C.. 1st Aid.. completing certain number of Weekends away, attends certain amount Thursday night Drill hall sessions. Were all typical examples of 'compulsory must does'. Warrants you a nice lump sum (sitting in your banks), each month of **April.**

Most our 'Bounty' was spent 'personal', on better equipment we treated ourselves trawling the Army Surplus Stores. Commercial Road So on.

Standard issue Army Kit you are issued with upon joining up only takes you, so far. So tarted up 'essential must haves list' benefiting our Soldering. Usually 1st thing to go was Dad's Army Helmets.

Exchanged in for better looking **Kevlar** Helmets. Lighter worn on long Patrols.

Bounty money wasn't too hard to earn. It was just great way making sure we knuckled down.

Army Weekends were ((once - every other week)), so most likely you'd fit in 2 Weekends away each Working Calendar month.

I want to see those Rifles spotless.

When finished cleaning our Rifles, Special Oil was rubbed on with the fingers, or a cloth, not to miss any small crevice, Weapons were always well Oiled.

The smell of Weapons was intoxicating, and I would usually get Home to say Mum & Dad, smelling of bullet rounds, weapons, Comradeship, Face paint, ((Camouflage)) or War paint.

Things that had gone off in Webbing, Rucksacks, a can of cola exploded, sandwiches ground in dirt, that only the birds tasted, in not wasting food. The Sun dried Mud, fresh & wet on our belly's, weekends over, was now solid.

Socks welded so hard, ((my boots taken off in relief)), they walked off on their own, crispy bang against the Wall Socks. My Mum would not appreciate these socks all my Army clothes, I was throwing off.

A good hot bath...

In with the other Laundry, not the wisest move, 'army clobber unthinkingly tired, went'.

These Smells, Actions I talk of, is more of those feelings you associate with Army. Like 15 years after leaving the Services exampled, you may pass a place you find yourself at with Smells sweeping in, ((that mind of yours, re-lives a place a position)) on earth, you were in the Army swept back. Thinks of those stirred up good times you had, Bonds you built.

Casting off many layers ((bubbles in your bath)), 'Matey Bubbles Smiling back at you', you jerk quickly half nearly fell asleep your overly-filled bath, pulling the Plug between your Toes, the 'Smiles' of gone good Memories.

Relaxing arms outside in my Radox bath, I was half head under water, ((un-winding the good memories I took back home with me)).

I was in possession of these Memories light, humour cast back, bath mirror reflections my reminiscing face, rubber ducking my bath water. No one in this normal World could see my memories ((gathered strength)), 'we all had as Soldiers', now taking in more bubbles, relaxed.

When gathering strength for our next venture Weekend away, a friendship built, the strangers you joined up with. In my case in ((Intake 5)), were now more than this. Still Happy in the Moment before our Next Weekend away, I remained cocooned in good thoughts only. Hoping I may make last this Great feeling, running like a buffalo's River through my Stomach.

They were my (left & right hand men), the good people I talk of, some cases women. They were my comrades, most of all they were my friends.

Working like this the; 'Way I do'. With my Asperger's. You might well say! 'you work so well with people Simon'. (Well true).

Though Simon who was a Carpenter in my day-job at the

time 'showed unfortunately **another persona**', to a job I enjoyed as Soldiering Simon.

Was easy in teamwork making friends, even with Asperger's I managed it. At a time was this that I thought I was normal.

You see in the Army was fun if you like camouflaged a hidden Asperger's roamer; a sleep I slept.

And not the Weirdo some were seeing in me 'Civilian life', a diagnosis not discovered yet.

I was built up, 800 people too all people I met. Trying to stay tuned into 'who I am'. Which led to struggles people rejecting the true me. I releasing often all 800 designer personalities. For the One person A.S. I protected.

Stated previously, my Works (Employment firm), didn't see Simon the Soldier which was my outlet a Hobby. They See Simon the Carpenter. Simon the he has his own mind Ideals. Then there was 'College boy Simon', who people again see.

Someone I was who would sit on their own. Sit at the front of the Class. Whilst others joked off, my willingness too learn. Participate.

Lunchtimes I sit on my own in Colleges refectory Halls Canteen. Feeling happy listening in; tannoy speakers wired above suspended ceilings. Playing Radio stations popular music. Used respective also 'info tannoy' College announcements e.t.c. While my other my Classmate Students filed off in Groupings I felt no Connections.

Sitting on my lonesome wasn't like this all times of course. I made, put myself out deliberately to sit 'with the main body of students' broken down groups encircled, familiarised in-breath College smells you, become accustomed.

The Voice in me; they shared no common ground, so mostly I sat there quiet unmoved.

Fortunately most often you find someone else as ((shy &

quiet)) as I was in those days', remains not so different today. That you may partner up with ((at dinner times)), so not looking that loose cannon. Marble runaway from pack.

My mood broke normality in the Routines, yet my mind ((wired to do well)).

Struggled through at times in College. At Work, out in the World. But never would I struggle in the Army, my best Colours came out. Left Alone.

This is where I came out 'my Shell', becoming a man/boy explains.

Forever I was changing costumes, to fit in - too be accepted.

Rebelled against criteria conformity, I felt it morally wrong loved, being loved, (by another, or a group), when you 'conform only' (to their fitting In).

If not a seen follow their Character 'their fashioned In' as a seen whole. Then you lost out, then you stood out. The ways not accepted straight away most often never. Passing energy that you said hey this is me.

Love another or group is 'power only your views', be objective. You had accept theirs the same.

I am reasonable understanding shall listen to another, this don't mean I want grow in his fitting. Friends won on fashionable personalities.

You see at a very young age I was showing signs of Asperger's already. Mixed in with good luck, normal Simon that could conform (dependant) Environment I found myself within.

Looking back over dig deep patchy memory. I find hard raise too a surface. Talking openly with you like this; does at least help my A.S.

A.S people respond well 'people show a', genuine Ace Card placed on Table.

That this friend says! 'you can trust my cards'.

A 'Follower' up-to ages 30ish - then I shed my follower qualities in for new Kit bags.

I was too 'lead'. I was Simon; the Leader. I was leading alright problem was I wasn't Leading others. I was Leading myself. Motivating myself. Pulling my own weights. Yet still others wanted Frameworks I wasn't born of.

I was becoming self sufficient, my boot heels were no longer dragging. This was at a time, I started Interested In Guitar. Year roughly 1998.

Trained myself in own Leadership, on Guitar.

I surrounded myself with Theory Books. Guitar Instructional D.V.D's. (Lick Library D.V.D's).

All bought from my benefits money. At times Labour Government were in Power. Tony Blair got in won 'three consecutive General Elections.'

Tony was Labours the UK's youngest PM since 1812. Although my understanding of it is: David Cameron took title (youngest PM since 1812) in 2010. Quite recent.

We had 10 good years of Labour (1997 - 07).

3 good years with our (Gordon).

Skins yellow.

My good friend John, carpenter A.E. Hadley's recruited me in T.A.'s. Also was a Corporal himself. Told me - take a look in his (bench draw) in work. 'One day'.

I did so being young, so easily came forward.

Opened this Wood swollen draw, wiggled it couple times, to get it open, and peered in. Copped!

He had **2** or **3** Banana **skins,** black bruised yellow he had left, with a green/ whitish colour exuding fungus white fur all over them.

Flies like (Blue bottles) large. Were flying circling the skins, in this draw.

Nearing heats of summer peaks. Where Factory windows doors commonly remained wide Open. 'Heats.'

Laughing his rocks off in his Union jack shorts. Seeing my stomach churn, full head of mine copped the worst hum of. Physically reaching expressions. He simply barrelled over in fits.

Unknown Autistic I was back in them days. I took it pretty well, (one) because he was my friend I always mucked about with him. (two) cause I can take a joke when it is meant harmless humour.

Looking back. (I break a smile) from time to time memories recited. At the genuinely harmless laughs. We all had.

Mouse in straw.

Another day at work in Hadley's this same Corporal, Carpenter bench joiner where I was working, I went up too him for our (little chats). I tendered to wonder often from my own bench area.

He had a **Shoe-box** in front of him one such day, from 'Clarks' I think.

He opened his Clarks' shoe-box 'White cardboard lid', inside was filled with yellow soft straw, like that on a Farm.

He said with a straight-faced honesty, put your hand inside Simon. So half wittingly, '**I thought OK.**'

Not knowing what to expect curiously reaching in, searching - I touched something softer than a Snake.

And in fact I thought it was a Snake. I moved the straw to one side upon inspection, to find he had only inserted a hole, just bigger than a **10 pence piece**, in the **middle**, the narrowest side of Shoe-box.

And what I grabbed hold of wasn't a Snake at all.

It was his D**k.

'**He creased up**'. A few of the other lads were rolling in stitches in all, killing themselves, it hurt to laugh in crying stitches. His actual first line to me 'is was' ((**do you** want to **see my mouse**)).

I thought he must mean a Mouse friend, like in the Green Mile, Mr Jingles. I guess this is what you call funny Sick Humour.

Hello Corporal.

((Stand at ease, stand easy Private Newell)). This was a greeting you 'knew now', what was to come next. **In the** ambiguous way **Corporal would sneak up** on us.

This meant as - there was a (tradition) that went around where someone was awarded, '**Shit-head of the day**'.

Or **King s**t.** (It happened to be my day), to carry this burden. Which was a plastic shit, probably bought from **U need Us.**

Where the Corporal would proceed, in opening the Private's, ((top right-hand - combat jacket pocket)), firmly leaving, **the deeds** with the **Private** stood too attention in front off him.

Upon this the Corporal then pivots an ((about turn)), **180 degrees** to the front, with a **smile on his face.**

And so signals the 'Private' ((he carries the weight of Problems, held by his Platoon)), freeing the minds of the fighting Soldiers, namely his combatants, his buddies, his Comrades.

Responsibility in **his** - left or **right**.. 'chest **pockets**'. In this case his 'top right pocket' (is left with him) - taking care of business, carries kept a good **Humour** our Platoon soldier when '**Moral**' was low.

Although this may seem wacky, you need Humour - certain ice-breaker if you are to Survive Army life.

Teenage turtle.

On another Occasion I was Crowned the most Wariest ba***rd (in Battalion), my Platoon.

Again this was Moral boosters people were gifted, half humouring rewards (given out) different ways, yet with an edge serious of thanking the soldier meaningful without thanking direct. Just suggestive - a man thing.

I Marched up to my 'Brigadier' at this time - I found myself In real man humanistic, balanced with authoritativeness temperament - he knew both lines sided disciplines his character when to switch it on, moderate reverse. He was the quiet helpful shadows, help in the field (high in Division), brigadier level. When the lads were down, missing their girlfriends back at home for example, he'd pep talk discernment care.

Brigadier swept in, wanted to reward me approve, my good works, hard fitness stealth keenly I showed, strength he see in me. I Saluted him (standing before the man), stepped back, adopting at ease position hands behind my back, head raised, tummy pulled In.

He after Saluted me, walked forward, placed in my possession on top of my head.

My beret he removed, a **Teenage Mutant Ninja Turtle Hat (Foam)** reefed in place.

This was acknowledgement notifying my effort-ed contributions rewarded as a way of a thank you, a little pat on the back, a well done you thing going on worthy of Brigadier wanting to thank me in some way. This was his way.

I thanked my Brigadier, ((about turned)) 180 degrees, walked off with a raised heartened **Smile on my face.**

At the Bar.

The Bar staff serving the soldiers (drinking room pub like) military bar facility, upstairs area Connaught Drill Hall building T.A Centre were brilliant. There was one particular man bar staff, 10 to 14 years my Senior, 'older in age.'

Had permed curly hair like Kevin Keegan - but tighter longer hair. So I'd say he was around 31 just by looking.

He was the person - we were thankful see. Smiling back at us, after a hard Weekend away, playing Soldiers. Pulling us a refreshing Pint.

Or as some say - playing Cowboys & Indians.

He made everyone bond without trying, feel the strength beloved, Army life talked, congregated soldiers nestled told Stories in. Sort of place you'd enjoy a good 4 to 5 pints, packing out close near (bar), standing tall very welcoming. Options reclining away soldiers en-grouped, engrossed sat around tables yearning a frothy realistic yarns talked.

This Bar person, **Bar staff** I talk of, reminded me of '**Joe Huff**' a character who goes undercover as '**John Stone**'. Fights in crowd gathered ring in the 1991 film '**Stone Cold.**' Played by 'Brian Bosworth' and Starring Lance Henriksen.

The barman I speaketh had (hard) - thumping out. A much good, solid standing character he lit presence, that it made you question wonder how one man might be both easily found. Our tall thin friendly Bar-man 'John Stone character' I described you.

We would sometimes, in a show of strength, I would be placed between **2 bar stools,** my army boots resting on one such stool, tip my head on another.

The rest of me was levitating in thin air.

Once ready I would shout for a **3rd Stool** grabbed by my left hand. Where I proceed to be counted jeered on for most amounts **Rotating** this not light **Stool,** around **my waist area,** as many times as humanly possible.

Competition popped hearts.

Walking away with say **50 turns** to **my name,** warmed competition on a first layer. My job then - **down necked 2 pints of lager.** 'I had mine with lime.'

I was unconventional, rather than direct Common. **Regal,** with a little easy- going pompous in me, beset seen might easily presume onlooking.

I proceeded into the next round **more Stool turning.**

And this is how it would go on, till enough was enough, taking seat back ((with the boys)), enjoying the Army Stories we shared, ordering the Rounds In.

In progressions night at the bar, shifting along, we had become a Family unit of people. Loving persons different people from different backgrounds, yet bonding (as one) this grandest room in/at the bar. Who knew each other like sister like brother, like strangers on joining up.

I should mention I was **Private Newell** upon joining up, given the nickname ((**TITCH**)), upon growth in my Career. I might have mentioned I was small joining this allegiance.

And what with Weight Training I done with Clive after Work, from job as a Carpenter. And what with carrying heavy, talking heavy **Back packs** in the **Army** for miles & miles to come.

And what with my friend **Steve West Thomas** - sometimes **Mark Ray,** Training with me In (Out of hours Army life).

I was like **little John,** who was big **called TITCH** with a Bicep you'd be Proud of.

Or as I once heard a college student say at College I attended in Bournemouth, ((**feel my Spuds**)).

Note: from Mum yet.

Always an (in-joke) 'with me/my Colour Sergeant', he would proceed in pushing my buttons.

Winding me up, which I took with a Humorous pinch of Salt.

'Private Newell,' he'd say: You got a '**Note** from **your Mother yet**?'

Referring to my baby-face child excitement. I brought keen along, now in a man's world.

This would happen every time we crossed Paths.

Cause small early quarters in of Army. I was a child very young looking at 17, so this was a hint at, you sure you're not lost or something, (baby school's the other way) was unspoken message Colour Sergeant spoke, with every got a: '**Note from your Mum yet.**'

I did find the funny side fortunately, he was someone ((I looked up to)). He knew, I knew he was (messing.)

And I knew he knew I took it as love comradeship, so a communication between just us, **breaking the ice, a man thing.**

Chicken on where! - the giblets.

On one Occasion in my Army Career, there was a Private 'Surname Largon' is all I knew him by.

He was from 1 or 2 Platoon, under his platoon commander Mr Griffiths, cannot remember names exactly.

Largon had got an erection, hard, like scaffolding poles, placed placing a medium sized Chicken, where one takes out the giblets.

Placed chicken bird all the way on ... I leave you to figure out where.

He than proceeded to run around the Drill hall swaying her left & right, commando. It was comical to say the least. Had us bursting out laughing.

My mum found this odd no wonder she thought, the Army was no good for me. A young mind I was at 17 was Immature. So I guess it is that time of Life thing we all do stupid things, Right? None more so than an admitting Immature happy Character I generally, looking back can see my errors. Yet all in all I felt safe in a daft World. Being liked had no attraction, had not exercised my escaping sensitive been, allowed to run VT.

Sunstroke.

Sun Stroke was a real threat on hot Summer days.

Or simply when yes it was hot.

We kept our Water hip flasks well topped up with clean fresh Water.

Some of our guys, the switched on ones at least, took energy boosting fluids to replace what the body was sweating out, stop people fainting by sides of the roads.

Or a wet t-shirt around the head, wasn't such a bad idea some might do both. 'Bathe'.

Wearing White clothing would help, wearing black clothing only attracts heat, whatever you did.

To lessen heatstroke affects, you took responsibility for advice is, in given. Though at the end of the day 'you are the Soldier'.

Most advice given had follow-through a chain of command, if you were not seen to be following orders, you would be given a 'show down'.

So although is your responsibility, take responsibility for your actions, had you not followed through with commands passed down, you surely would have been dressed down.

I guess those above you know best.

Regardless, everything should be tested. You as a Soldier could have come up with the newest ways in preventing sunstroke, (by going against command), cause people are not testing (as you do), they are quite correctly just obeying.

You see, what I mean by taking responsibility then for your own actions.

The way Asperger's find holes in many Theories he is firstly shouted down, then congratulated later, for all reasons he went against command, to obtain lost information useful to him.

'Now you', who were quick to dis-believe, quick to obey **is not wrong**, ((in fact your doing the right thing, the neutral that is right in safety)). However,

had such great scientists/Inventors obeyed man's fit in demands followed ((all laws)) of try and tested, then people such as **Nikola Tesla**, American Inventor

Electrical/Mechanical engineer 'a future visionary', might have missed out on Inventions, won congratulated achievements.

One such invention discovery, his known best ((he/we, could of lost out too)), was the designed ((Alternating Current Electricity **A.C.**)) system supply, he contributed to man's excellence.

Then where would we be? '**Up** the **creek without a paddle**', had it not of been for the brilliant pursued mind that is Nikola.

Nikola had his fair share of people disbelieving in him. A.S. absolve this common faultiness the hurdles in his own mind, our mind met with a fair amount of conflict and challenges. He would need override if only he was to stay on path. His own deduced calculations; trusting in his theories.

He was also taken advantage of throughout his life, or more to the point 'the ideas patented to him', were in many ways if you like stolen by others, claiming rewards from the hard work that is Nikola.

Despite; he rose above many sometimes doubting people he endured. Since his quest was driven to better man's knowledge. At a loss to his own routines he'd require a high discipline.

Obtaining results from harmonised 'hypotheses' conducted by free flowing energy. Nikola depicted his in/out positives & negatives a batten of seen advances working progresses. Towards nailing hard evidence secure believe in his hunches his theories his suspecting conclusive theories rounded up. Only he lived in this world. That would eventually give way to life of Wireless Radio as one of many exponents. He worked on from driven believe.

Like Nikola Autistic man (fought life) theory based uniquely his. This is what it means to be Autistic.

Autistic is a man wanting his own World. Space to work.

Many dedicated hours day & night he slaved practical experiments. With no guarantees his workings would show light. He gambled this against his own self-believe the assumptions he continued to bring around as laws of principles. That stood competition out the water.

The fact is, like many Great minds through History he had the self believe (he alone ran with). Breaking through to a believe set of principles, he kept hypothesizing, going going going, with many disappointments, he wasn't swayed. Much like A.S. obsess a driving force.

He knows, questions answers that drove him 1st obsess; he just requires a time space enveloping existence. True truth hunches behind his hungry thirsty his fingers at work come-by 'a proven work'. Tweak add diminish, all **standard scaled models** we keep as home bases. So never lost in a return. The Lab models aiding his visions put too ground.

'The mind that is you' till daylight shines. A 'Sundial'. Pass cast awaited. Awaiting a shadow your physical energy.

All possible set working conditions. Meeting said 'mad scientists' life style. In similar fashion A.S people must hum a harmony. Conditioning. Custom mind cares. His concentrations housed.

Funding available to all. The naked we came into the world penniless. Garments of the finest fabrics matters very little unfolding; without permissions granted.

Butterflies driving home. Interests you chase rationalizing. Pay off is healthy heart in sync, not snagged under disbelieve.

Autistic A.S. like Nikola must Isolate into a loneliness a private communication. 'Harmonium mind' my friend. ((The quiet voice friend)). You tap a wavelength vibrating; most in a normal world find wow that is amazing. Yet for us satisfaction mustn't stop - extra doing well.

We want to obsess much more 'yet like Nikola' require make a surviving living. Nikola not reliant on others, (**his dream like A.S.**) was lock himself away find general Interests untested. Strange Interests palette of principles 'hypotheses', driving him come up with solutions satisfaction not resting in him. Showmanship worthy he or I reach a point ((worthy)). Expectations thirsting solutions he must Work like A.S. no matter not granted.

Asking less of a man freedom, that you are freedom gave you freedom.

Autistic people like Nikola Tesla are/were a (Patent) that can't be copyrighted.

T.A. to Police force.

A lot of the Army Officers from the T.A Units includes Regulars I believe, joined the **Police Force**, going from a Soldier to Policeman.

Was sort of a transition thing that went on. The background you came from, be this T. A. or Regular Army, ((thinking in a Military disciplined way)), gave you a foundation easier to lay down, adapt into, when making transition from Army, to Police Force.

This was a transition phase, step - I heard a few do.

Gave a Refreshing break some will crave, to his **New phase in life**, now as **P. C.** someone.

In the Army you was never given time to think. It was get your Scram (Food), down your Necks, that's how it would go on. **On the double.** Everything had to be done yesterday, this was a help and a hindrance rolled In one neatly folded blanket, depending on the mind that was you.

Walking from Home - to T.A. Centre.

Walking from my Home meeting at Army T. A. Centre for your Weekends away, Thursday night drill or visa the versa contrariwise - walk bus car - back, you felt overawed.

I, on Occasions depending, made my journey was dressed like a Christmas Tree, Dads' army. I was anything but camouflaged, blue skying urban city, my greens in civilian's chivvy world before arriving at TA Centre on time safely.

Looking camouflaged, like one in scrim nets, heavy baggage, dads' army helmet lid clang, clanging. Metal buckle things sway symbol-ed rhythm. Every stranger out in public ((looks)) reigning me dry I walked effort-ed exerted steps.

I must have looked a right sight, like the Mr Friendly smelly man. Every city has one.

Getting on Provincial buses/double deckers barely reaching 'change' pay driver my ticket. Turning knocking people my spade poking out.

People with eyes fixed on me, screwing their faces up, rose noses up that they did look like the back end of a bus.

In the Army you got use to the grouching, encroaching uncomfortable, people stares around you, giving you uncomfortable energy to move along with.

We forgave, forgot you brushed the dust off Soldiers' - Shoulders.

Puffed up your little chest bigger, fought through harder.

Asking the 2nd Opinion.

I asked someone once what do you think of me as a Soldier in Army, although Asperger's I wasn't aware of at this time.

It mattered to me, to ask others what they thought of me, once in the while.

The guy I asked was probably, 'less liked than I'.

So seeing as I got more attention than him, and was quite popular, a little more than him - I thought I'd ask the one who would, how can I put it, be more jealous of me.

Although the way I word it, it isn't as harsh as jealousy.

But it's the best I can do, 'so work with me'.

He said: you're a little too enthusiastic, a little too longing thirsting attention to be the best from my seniors above me, a little too much not from the quoted real world he was from.

Of course he didn't say this per word of tongue, though his - dropping a spanner in works language gave you word unspoken.

I lived in a fantasy world, where I thought everyone was good in the World, perhaps because I only lived in good ways.

Perhaps why I was one of the fittest in my Platoon, at the time, I had the fitness strength, and strong moral, pushed on in me drive, with the kindness you think I am.

When others were dropping out - flaking to the gutter, I had an ingredient extra they were lacking it would seem. Love was my strength, loved by others made me work harder. Was this so wrong? Apparently so.

So Asperger's or not. The person I am, through felt love I felt I was receiving, was as much of the so-called real World I wanted ditched, unless espoused purported my first simple gift first adaption persona smiling along, pleased with my lot.

So you see, being an outstanding Soldier, I was pleasing some, and through no fault really, making others, shall we say, Jealous, or maybe Envious. Words evaporated cream in my walk walks best.

The **person** I asked his **2nd Opinion on me**, Informed me, in so many words, I was...too 'keen', too 'excited', too 'Enthusiastic', too wanting all the Special attention. Then you hear that **Government's People's people** you meet on Journey throughout life say: it's this shared enthusiasm we are looking for **in another Voice.**

Contradictory I took on board, mixed messages left voiced come Normal people, come Aspergers people. Damned if do, damned if we don't. Worldly message, not matching regular shout, (snap). 4 Kings, 4 Jacks won.

Guitar life/Army life.

My Guitar life, my Army life.

I see me as: '2 very different people'. My Army life was active. I was projecting the real Simon, who just wanted a career in Army, to be loved as a Soldier.

My Guitar life, which started what I don't know - 14 years after I first began my Army career at aged 17, was when I was in my 30s.

I had felt the Reality of life by now, what with the knocks life ((gives you)), was very shy, introverted, recluse, gone back in my shell. As I'm sure many are though (echoed in Asperger's), with more, much more, amplification turned up inside him. Shows me.

That is when I found an Interest for guitar, in Mill House, a hostel I stayed.

A friend called 'John Thompson', he'd got me started on Guitar, just learning a few simple 'riffs' such as:

Smoke on the water, (Deep purple). Eric Clapton riff, taken from a song called: Sunshine of your Love.

In the getting me started, John took distraction away an otherwise outside bustling World gearing unwanted predictable pressure. John's help helping me, friendship my friend John Thompson, offered.

I already enjoyed the arts to Philosophize before Guitar life, in my head in general.

So Guitar Theory Guitar Practice, had me asking lots of Questions, not all Guitarists themselves could answer, you just had to assume, move on.

I guess that's what divides one guitarist from another, what creates the Interesting tensions in music, music gives us.

So I treated my Guitar as if it was Human, this Box with a **hole in middle body**, the Neck 6 strings.

My Acoustic 'had become an extension of my Arms. Hands.

Fingers'. My brain gave signals Hands, Fingers, then Strings. Then gave me information back, a Sound I told it to perform, strings back to Ears.

So when you hear persons having a Relationship with their own Guitars, this is not far off mark.

I became to philosophize in Guitar Theory.

Shuttled my own self away from the Society I thought I knew, person I was in the Army, was now nothing more than memories I couldn't trust, only seen swimming an empty shell. I was lost for the golden truth, knocked confidence

the stinger removed from my rattle. Found a peach easily in confidence before, the pre-date mentioned. My A.S Colouring book started too fill.

Looking back later on in life, I wonder how I could have been so strong, so able to be confident, though I will say this confidence again, was due with me thinking everyone loved the same as I do, not knowing any difference, I'm different.

It was like back in the day 'of well-liked Simon'. I had a Guardian Angel over- seeing those trying Shadow an awkwardness in me, I wasn't of then.

Was naive, more so younger, not understanding those get got angry with me, was resilient to fight off my not understanding others yet gullible, a sucker punch to keep peace. Those not fully coming as the glowing friend, wolves in sheep's clothing, friendly Nature, pure in Spirit. Yes, was all I knew.

My Conscience back in the day of happy free - Spirited Simon, the real Simon was (not awakened Consciousness), how the real World operated.

My cotton wool I was wrapped In, was of a Special kind, angered those to the playful Spirit I was. So had I upset anyone by the real Simon, who I really was, (than I was protected in thinking my actions were of the Normal). Why I might have been treated the same.

Why perhaps others were not understanding me, treating me in the so called Normal genders, to an otherwise Asperger's still awaiting a diagnosis.

Down in a frown.

I was now walking my own paved path in life.

So I was now Obsessed with Guitar, I cut all communications with outsides World - for over 12 over 14 years, still am this person today for reasons I was frowned upon.

For reasons my in past growing ups, when was happy I was energetic. I retreated somewhat instead home philosopher.

I was at this transition in my life anyhow, had I been happy or sad. I found I was at a cross junction, much like Robert Johnson the Blues player, who came

to a cross roads, selling his soul to the Devil, in history I read with Interest, gone by.

Becoming grey Simon not speckled, people I met would wonder why I was not happy, full of same charisma juice, they enchantingly ladled, or I once was.

Maybe I just was looking maladjusted reasoning comfortable in place, reversing what Normal identified as. My break different, difference A.S. safety net.

Looking at me obscured, a buttoned-mouth of Words, no longer coming through Customs. Words non releasing in me like Chinese lanterns as a Normal should, and why I was now seen as Weird Simon.

I was Aspergic before my division. Guitar life and in Army life/family life there wasn't a point ever I wasn't Autistic you would assume, just unknown.

Family life was a ((loving environment)), so one may assume this was a peak where (A.S slept unseen), yet I'm sure talking too my brothers, sister, parents family visiting they'd disagree. So if love was an anti-dope reducing seen Autistic Simon - then this was the one exception to the rule.

Yet the Army was given me 'the born love' my asperger's didn't show up in.

'Had I not this love'. I believe I'd have had a Diagnosis 'seen in me earlier.'

All I understood was, without a Love surrounding me, Asperger's Syndrome heightened my crumbling self.

After army life, I saw the cold-shoulder of life, which I'd never experienced in my naive life up to this point.

What with the 'drug taking' in my life now, replacing natural love.

Unashamedly, because the ((love was missing)). I was dosed up on cold shoulder fluids 'the world had shown me', from run corn wrapped up in cotton wool person I started out as. So showing a 'not caring Simon', was my best chance of protection now. Hey, if people leave you alone when you're miserable as Sin, not a problem I'll do this too.

Becoming now this Guitarist, who was loving his Guitar only, for fear of the outside World, and how cruel it can be, so literally I thought playing Guitar, will escape me from those not wanting to see me as I am. When, all shields of protection are allowed to drop, the preferred Simon I'd have rather been.

So much like before the dragging affects of others repressing me, was still not accepted (by them) in me, for me showing suitcases of happiness love, which I deemed as the only way to be.

So a Resolution was not Resolved in me, nor tried make me feel happy as I am.

My Asperger's laid dormant like a Cancer in me, ((never seen before)). I though feel A.S. was in me coming through, my said devised Normal interrupted, not left alone.

At a phenomenal express train rate begged a belief 'not Logical', when AS was said seen or when Simon said was Normal.

Though A.S. was ((not a word known)) I heard so much before, turning doors before welcomed Millennium. 20th Century gone. 21st said hello.

Especially now: I felt pressured hiding the real me, feeling a safety benefit army/home-life provided. 'I required operate on.'

Disregarded one minute, looked up to the next. Had Asperger's **showing quicker** - times disregarded and times suspension praised was left! from transparent dominant A.S towards; dormant translucent cloudy seen Asperger's, my drug influenced world reality jobbing dogged me extra unaided.

Interest I function normal on, is asked condition's flower arranged, arranging my way.

My flesh on bone is a candle lit as (Normal Simon) seen by you. Thriving on conditions I ask, A.S sleeps, granted all my conditions met laid plans, breaking an A.S.'s code agitates his conditions brought on.

Thankfully I left a little mist to my own transparent Asperger's window, so cloudy A.S., and why I am Mild Asperger's.

It is possible I may make loss soon 'my **Mild title**', very soon gone, I will one day be augmented '**fully Aspergic.**' I feel it weighing on me in Waters, that a re-diagnosis may give me my **new** disorderly **prognosis.**

The confident young boy ((society wanted to see)), it was assumed, ((had people jealous of him, jealous of me)), who people didn't like seeing this confidence in me!

They were jealous I reckon. I didn't function a beat of their drum, was even told by a former friend. He said Simon, I'm jealous of you.

I respected him though straight for telling me.

I had a strength 'he liked', though rather embrace my friendship his best intent was destructive, he couldn't articulate so he stole installed a brokenness in me.

I wanted him to feel the confidence I was feeling.

Brought up in a sheltered life where I was only taught love & goodness running through my veins - was this so wrong?

I thought this, my goodness, open envelope was what every person felt. If it wasn't and said I am not of a real world, then I marvelled, wherefore thunder clapped happiness unslammed unbullied my way gave rise statistics an open real World photographed. One perfect picture abidance only advocates their support flimflammed right.

The problem was, he, my jealous friend, wanted to show me his world, while I was wanting show the good, **I rehearsed by him**, and so it felt like a test, of him swallowing me up, running me by ((challenging ways too my good strong strength, I thought I had)). Coming out other side, seeing if my **Weebles Wobble but they don't fall down** ((a toy from 1970s)).

Bounced up as strong. Something no one should test friends don't do that, they know the result untested. The jealousy ways he injured exhausted on **my good me** with no wobble, the one I preferred, wobbled breaking me in open waters of his real world.

I was not accustomed or strong to break my own falls 'he see, he knew' (**stood lights - my character**), was taken in his world of sink or swim. If I was, then so it was taken advantage of ((gradually over time)), till his mission was complete. He achieved what he came to break in me forever, after which his uses for me absorbed away the fragile **protective coatings - I once was bound confident**, you might say naively.

I never did understood people who got angry. I do now a days of course, because I became this angry person 'others were' shown as asperger's, my aspergic way.

So what did I do? I swapped my Rifle for a Guitar: reflective of good and bad governments.

I swapped drugs somewhere for Innocents.

I swapped easily distracted and became strongly principled, reverting through back and forth distractions.

I swapped: my guard down - and took my made mistakes.

This list above: non stop (adds) no end a pen run dry. Ink already circular ongoing universe. Expanding, shrinking constellations, known unknown. A.S found with rejected (drop hat) lost moments.

When this, my transition ((set dividing lines in me)), I was becoming a very 'not nice Simon'. An out of Character Simon, an Aspergic Simon cloudy.

Therefore not A.S Normal good Simon.

Showing a quietened down Asperger's I had. ((Showing more transparent clean window)).

Stirred waters showed: cloudy A.S. Murk - left alone settled clear waters.

This nasty, confused, less balanced Simon, was playing still beautiful music on his guitar, good nasty up and down orchestra of feelings testing as human, you call this as you will. Was spearheaded with many incoming advances, explaining dogging many moods Autistic man 'known, unknown I was' let slip that's not what I mean so much.

I'm discussing the **reserved me** at times I was playing Guitar a: **reversal mood** said **seen.**

Was my drug taking my way of fitting in as Normal? Though closer to numbing (the different I was), I pretended to be this guy Normal I wasn't.

My drug taking surely induced a heightened Autistic conformation my bright (star), seen against black sky at night Simon's delight.

Governments not of Labour did bearing heavy: The Normal I tried mixing as, a confirmed Autistic in manner: I couldn't become something just cause a switching of governance ordained a World whipped their shapes heavily reigning, the man of Spectrum freely conditions his conclusion different non- conformist.

An adjustment I accepted, for new peace quietening of mind. One beneficiary slides good, yet losing my happy other beneficiary self.

So people would easily blame my Guitar - my Army life, maybe even my College - my Work Employment life for my said bad attitude bar-graphed strangely with good attitudes, keeping log books simply gave no logic.

Sometimes you could argue strong, sometimes you could step away from your own conclusion the Aura of temperaments I purported your way as your seen truth. Truth true was, depending on the changing days I was In, and what shading Autistic gave Normal as today.

Now I don't want you thinking:

OK so you only had Asperger's when you left the army, cause more than likely it was there as a **wrist band on me** in the **army**, ((yet wasn't 'fluorescent' in the **dark**)).

Therefore, a love provided I once did know hid my asperger's - in Army Green.

Drugs my own path foolishly I now wanted to walk ((without the confidence)). I wished was there, without a love running through my veins, replacement 'showed you Hubble telescope on' **where** my Asperger **lived** highlighted.

I'm not saying either: I am not Aspergic with love!

I most likely am, just less detectable my A.S. Is, when (Asperger's normality), swims freely **with love in trunk.**

Incredible Hulk.

It is just like the; Incredible Hulk. Where the radiation he was exposed too. Brought out a Character in him that couldn't be seen when, people were nice to him.

When the Hulk was ((gotten mad)) gotten Angry. He was showing green Asperger's in comparison.

And now, you could see in comparison with me his 'Heavy Green Colours' of my Asperger's.

Mild A.S is 'light shades of green' he swollen up as ((a comparison my own mild A.S. light army greens)).

He was (The Hulk) '**before he'd gotten mad 100%** also an inner green tempered dormant Smile expected of fit in; light to dark Autistic man.

You can philosophize on what I've told you say well if, you was this before/this now **than why** at **one stage** of your **life,** had your Asperger's turn coated sporadic Light and sporadic Dark Greens.

I can only make you one Interpretation for what it is, ((time spaced on Writing I am)).

As I stated my case and why misunderstanding in others (tells you usually) why you misunderstood for he has, ((Aspergers Syndrome don't you know)).

Asperger's is my natural language. We see as right for us. I cannot step away change. Hence I am Autistic orientated.

Take what I say as an accepted truth mine I work within, please.

Asperger's I am about 'Non changement'. Cannot change actions I display. Tells you why my found diagnosis. Is me.

Fix bayonets.

Well OK then.

In the Army Fixing Bayonets. ((A Knife locked into, 'Rifles end of barrel' **bayonet stud**)).

Was used for close range killing, should you be Mr unfortunate 'running out of bullets'.

Or you have yourself feed jam - won't clear.

Than fixing your bayonets, may be your only wisest move left.

Attaching a 'Knife' end of rifles snub, gives the **extra extension**, strength, leverage, taking your enemy out quietly. Or running them through, at them like a crazy man.

Body beautiful.

Back in days of my body beautiful, looking at my well formed forearms whilst weight training.

Curling dumbbells, Curling bars. **The pump** the weights gave you.

Was something else. **Mirror poses.**

Pumping up biceps, triceps, laps, crunching abs, was like drug natural, best form. Staring back at me in Mirror reflex.

Whilst exchanging arms in dumbbells, my bending in ((repetitions)) had my '**wrist watch**' casting **Shadows.** Spots beaming a narrow torchlight moving up down ceiling to walls, then back walls to ceiling.

Intrigued by the moving circle of light given by '**Sun shining** in a top louvre Window' the pauses in weight. Taking a breath, much like music breathes, you see training light dot flickering, stopped to the pauses.

My 'Watch' on hold, hear faint tick.

Weight training, loving yourself in body beautiful, is why others will love you. My 'dot' back on the move A.S. fun.

Army Chapter 8 ends. Halts.

Chapter 9

Jason & the Argonauts.

'A great film called' **Jason** & the **Argonauts,** reminds me of when the **'GODS'**, ended the Games they played with Jason. Saying in a language there will be more adventures, and challenges for Jason.

The games they played with **JASON** they'd had their fill. 'Saying JASON will - have his day', **too come out fighting** when the GODS set 'New Game & Times.'

Jason for now, **will build** in the **Wins.** His already taken back. Will be thankful for his 'gains'. 'His' influences gave better arguments Jason battled hard. **Rests better** each time. **More battles** are **Won.** 'Losing to Win' in the now rest his seeking.

Rest Jason 'the GODS demanded', a closing.

Come on - you can tell me.

Normal acting, seen **Autistic man.** Is people working **with him** his relaxed self. You can't guarantee his kept conditions shall remain (environment Works). Made from a Ton of non conformists too his ways.

Even when people are nice too us they may hide what makes us both connect. So I am at a loss again.

I always preferred my life walked alone. For I am in flagrant I carry; my own reassurance uninterrupted.

I Don't keep 'middle road growing optimistic opinions' your conclusion made half judging 'Alternative thinkers' distant **poor vision** like an **elephant** is better smarter. Only information forth coming at him come closer dim the lights ((do you see))? Strong understanding.

Had I swam all reasonable information of, the quality we are talking about 'eye sight that of the Elephants' would have, seen **sharper than** a Tooth Necked Saber Tiger.

Are you willing **change** too **another Side** on the whim **every time** you have **new thoughts.** Or do you just support The favoured football team exampling, never love other teams. ((Cause you already in this team)). Setting your precedents a magnet you cannot change. Answering Yes you cannot change indicates you my reaction of (change) ensued on me enlarged. Tells you why I cannot Change. I am what I am. In this case an A.S man.

Issues to my, A.S. satisfaction.

Is there **a difference** in me saying to you, look **can I Volunteer** ((said simply, work for my benefits)) **in love** do able **results** whilst you carry on splitting hairs, ((to what is acceptable)). Serving the Community under thumb nails heavy hand.

Distributing **Lib Dem** leaflets one angled example. Discussions talked on in previous.

Some receiving my leaflets might screw up, throw away in the **waste paper basket**, the same as I do with **Pizza Menu's** & other **Junk Mail** I receive.

Wasting yet more paper, even though I pasted front door...please!

'**NO JUNK MAIL** PLEASE'. '**NO CIRCULARS**'. '**NO MENU 'S**'.

Leaflets posted. People continue using Junk leaflets ((as **shopping lists**)), or a reminder to the boyfriend not too forget to feed the dog, **they write** for **themselves on** the **backs** leaflets.

Costing affect wasting leaflets paper pulped from trees not, cost effective man hours, of our precious Taxpayer crying a lumber-jacking his ham and mustard sandwiches a days works. I letterbox post money forked out.

Walking out in a few communities. I felt no welcomed message feeling apart of people. Simply, **I'm not apart of them**, remain **nice nature, soft weak.**

Broken who I am my conduct way I explain I carry myself. Including my A.S same Cousins. Not really ever happy stay out side ((in community - for too long)). I walk back Home writing my feelings down with you.

Caring compromise is rare. Reasoning to assert my better **position with you,** will be **slammed down** obscure **every time,** ((by you)), like an 'American footballer' tackled sending out messages his World. Restless **care** 'the **Values.**'

Care Compromise we follow merry go a rounds. 'Tells you', I'm not like you. I am 'Asperger Syndrome'.

My Doctor's said same **found** the **diagnosis in me** challenged thinkers all A.S.s, fight good challenged fights.

People often said Simon, I can't find nothing wrong with you, ((you've **heard me** say this **before**)). Yet when the idea's I culminate too 'are lesser **thought ways,** I assumed'… it is then my symptomatic awkwardness says hello. Systematic diagnosis **shown in all** Asperger's following the Spectrum.

I met a lot of **Asperger's people,** that **don't** want to be! **Aspergic any more.** Trying too remove their, '**Labels**' of **Asperger's** in what I see as unwise. Unclicking 'your Seat-belt', whilst belting it down Motorway won't work for you.

Since when 'you did' try **change back** become **NORMAL** 'cause you were told this is what most people think you are' ('**it didn't** work, **for you**').

So I say too you. When Doctors & Professionals above me **gave me my diagnosis,** it was through years of Study (they are Qualified In). In the trust we ask them for, **help leading us** too our **right prognosis.**

I was even **accused once, I hide** behind my **diagnosis** yet, when I came from outside of the Curtain **they,** couldn't **lead me** in ways **I have** always **worked** still seen as Asperger's.

Because it's these lengths **all Asperger** people **go-**

to (if not appreciated Listened too) set formation he contingently continues asked.

Is why **you see** some Autistic whose had proper Diagnosis, **trying** too **deny** this **part of them.** Like visiting a Tattooist then not liking your Tattoo.

Now claims to your skin ((show Asperger's)). **'A tattoo,** I am not **ashamed In**'.

Oh no not Voluntary again.

Other Voluntary Jobs I'm willing work my benefit in is, Computer Data input, you've heard me say. My step dad Paul first gave me this Idea.

You can sack your Secretary's, let Simon do your Inputting.

Meaning you no longer have to pay a weekly wage too the **employed Secretary,** 'you fancied for years', ((but is saving you money letting her go)).

When you can (get out of) **Work Benefit Volunteers** doing the same job **for free** 'for you'.

An A.S man is heavy encumber-some. Go against him you see Mental illness faster than most. Closing him down. (Lift him up) you see A.S man performing faster than most.

We may ask you for our own **cap badges** sat in **our berets.** Known simply as: 'The Benefit Volunteers **Badge**'. Asperger Red colour.

Bit like **The Salvation Army Badges.** They proudly wear.

We shall no longer be known '**dirty dozen, benefit claimants**', we shall be seen in new lights. Same as a **Skoda Car** was seen **in a bad light.**

Recent years! The Skoda Car is: '**Bentley Rolls Royce** of Cars'.

Hans Lecter.

I require to be left in a job ((where I'm on my own))

same as Hannibal Lecter lived on his own. In the film The Silence of the Lambs. And had his Drawings looked after by Barney Matthews.

((Head Orderly at Baltimore State Mental Hospital)).

He bargained for more 'throughout the film' a Window with views (to a Wood) he can see through. Then one week a year on Plum Island, beach walks/ swims on an Island. Dr Lecters reward F.B.I. he helps. Save Catherine Martin... his open Sea Air, privileges.

Where his mind truly gifts him... a peaceful place philosophy unfold no restrictions his good works he wanted at performance level.

Voluntary Work is my preferred option. I am taking **up** with the **Job centre.**

Chapter 10.

Asperger's are the learners only. In their 'One only' chosen Subject.

Asperger people don't work in quote: full capacity Full time Job (The - well). Particularly my noted reported association no connection uninterested robotic love. Cause Asperger are the 'Learners', how might they Learn if they are (Working)? how should can they function obsessed too an Interest. Of their eggs all in one basket own?

You may say actually I know my friends Mums daughter who is Autistic. And she's one of the best workers in her factory. I sure hope this is the case this is encouraging I'd reply. Yet by & large Asperger persons remain Awkward in Communication stubborn. Don't want too mix generally they wish mostly stay in Communication they obsess. His Worlds protects Walls Shutters Up.

His mind spindle moulds 'the directions he holds', his mind just for you air free makes expansions, ((worth his while)). This to an Aspergic person is a healthy Sea breeze, he'll demand a Condition. Pointing out every step way the over explanations **dragging him down** a moulded road not of him never wanted never holding focus.

'Then when forced', down roads not of his choosing, his made fun of... (cause guess what), he just don't fit In. Then the arguments start again they might say Simon, I don't get it, you seem so normal.

Treated like Normal follows next, meaning I'm fake smiling back at people, I'm back again living up too this Stony Beach I find hard a tread with no shoes no socks on. People are looking at me strangely, an awkward Normal terrain I traverse - beach pebbles & flints cutting into Asperger's I was diagnosed with.

Asperger people absorb Information like a Sponge, they shall have **One Specialized Way of Learning.** They persist in a Subject, they can't stop talking about, **'mine was Guitar'.**

Asperger like **'New' Learning** Introduced as ((small saplings)). Time in growing... Non push for example.

An Asperger person starts learning about things like: The **Braking Systems** of a **Car**, about old brake disc systems, should he purse/pertain to this subject. **As his** given **subject loved.**

Learners of: Car Breaking Systems Asperger person ((**in Obsession**))... chooses topics subjects ((as so)), **bore** the **pants off most...** in this case 'Car Braking Sys'.

Yet **these Obsessive Interests** he religiously marries himself into...begins off as the Learner, **in his** chosen **subject...**then becomes an Owner, ((his new book)) called: **'Braking Systems'** The overlooked/underlined. Troubleshooter. Made easy for average Car Owners.

My Newest Compulsion is 'Writing books' my old compulsion playing Acoustic Guitar/Electric Guitar, due **stages my life** I'm In.

My compulsions for writing books may seize one day though, what control running me away can I decide my future?

I guess fascination builds loves an admiration for people uncertain, their world around A.S, our certainty is built first then broken... nothings ever quite yours.

Through a **fearful World,** you never quite unfold a person, 'you like' person (another makes you).

It is hard to know where you might find an Author of a Book that resides a message in you also, you take a sigh of relief your message spoken.

A seedy leafy Bar down the narrowest street is one such Authors Home. Namely mine.

The best Authors...! oh people you hate the most, **'person people,** you gave all your evil stares too, through

- out your years'... the ones you pass on streets.

Those you felt they trash... were the ones in-fact you should have thanked, respected, while life was passing by you. Surely.

Next time go out in the World. Try adjust your attitude please, too all people you feel anger towards 'with no real reason to as to why' **you just** don't like **him her.**

Then **think** what if his **got Asperger's**? He hasn't his Normal... then considerate towards your fellow man people **you for** no reason **hate,** should be where you make ((Key Change)).

Turning you a decent human-being, you was once.. but have gotten lost through life's tangles, as we all do, (from **by them** whom forcefully you were, **led too follow**).

This is your chance tell yourself not too late make, your difference.

All people we meet.

Not just select hand few here there, 100% adjustment.

Love you show message passed too another person.

When your peers, ((see this as a rightful thing do)), not a joke piss take thing do.

Your army of strengths, shall domino affect message is honest passing not, you following no more, but you leading.

This is your Chance.

This is your chance turn it around, (Smiling) everyone who passes you by out walking, in your car, on bus, in a taxi, on a plane...also passes (your smiling strength on). Freeing you up jobs got on with. We know how good you are, why do we know, how might we know?

We're love of you ((not dissing you)). Person I am is everything you allow form mould take shape. Is firstly cherubs persons' run **same high.** Respects you give yourself returned.

Simply I like you Weak Poor/Rich Strong Famous, famously Infamous, liked unequivocal same respecting. Rich and Poor I like to show I am both and took one. Untiringly up & down in a graph wavering. Taking it on the chin accepting all experience survivable freedoms you set. You see Autistic lines are never static... never in equilibrium... so look **enjoy.**

Not so fortunate under privileged Children & Adults, alike equal not better than Richer Wealthier kids/ adults. Vice versa appeal return home. Both Classes **merger of one.** Not minding when one which follows or in what order. Not minding roles you bag for yourself in life's journey is true wealth experience you bagged on travel, 'thanks rich & poor people' a same gratitude.

Of course bad language found, scrappy manners found... be you poor or rich 'is not no' commodity a step forward. Where poor and rich bond friendships grow paralleled. No jealous.

Such dreams I recite World... effort helps turn.

Treating considered stupid people we never met before, with an assumed Intelligence we gave them. ((They the A.S or ill informed)) found that all forms of Intelligence however praised up, looked down never was an Intelligence wider Community's, World in general all gave back. Regarded Normal N.T.s favouring a Normal class higher he/she unconsciously not meaningfully see Normal people as the Master race.

Bigots full of own cream is a quick reaction Autistic man mistakes his mumbles with some Normals he ingests.

You might say Aha Aha... half my friends are Normal... half my friends are Autistic functioning. Though I personally haven't found this true and when is true It is possible ((through the Smiles)), a battle quiet can tell smell my Autistic Persona. Giving Aura not supplementing Normal Circles input.

Not respecting awareness '**Unwanted s**' in Society bigoted of man crumbled. Fell to dust fall out my A.S. Cousin's hand.

It is us Autistic declaring now shall suck up our Cocktails on Islands only imagination 'frees thoughts' free of damnation release part paves non knotted.

Fondness Intelligence ((brokered into)) **Unwanted s** showed them as, smart Intelligent.

Not taking them the fools, welcome accept no one is above another - we once were told, (if he is saying) fun intelligence he believe he **hadst.**

Is **hadst only** when I giveth same respect too others, (I gave me.... **hadst... had**).

You know just of how much warmth you can keep 'goodwill'.

Loving more every passing second (Glow your Love). Like Holy Spirit around you. Speaks his or her Words... **by so**, you are happy free running through me (the sound of shackles removes).

Happiness I am for you, now you '**In me**'… passes to you.

Happy my face glowing, mirroring shared appraisals twisted butterflies in stomach smile going forward. **I am - you** unshackled.

Life path number 8.

My Life Path Number is **8.** In a Numerology sense.

Here's a Chart that explains me Simon I was given. That I thought was very accurate. This Chart I've logged further on, turning pages.

Take look further on.

Simon **With** & **Without** Asperger's is a person **I am.** In this Chart 'before & after Diagnosis'. And was still this the same person.

I just had more to-go on is all **when** Diagnosed **Aspergic.**

All my unanswered questions! Made a lot more Sense. It was a Sword fish speeding through the ocean **meeting up** with my **new founded diagnosis** not so alone. I had the schooling of other Sword Fish close by forming closing In.

Jumping out under deep majestic dark turquoise blues lives, ton set heavy waters. Landscaping bodies of Ocean liquid bursting sun glint blue Waters happiness. I finally belonged to a group of Sword Fish rarely seen together. Before **diagnosis** I was **lost,** a Sword Fish migrating a wanted roaming answers my questions.

A.S. Is... **'A. S.**word fish'. A likeness founded In me I had, a category now Swordfish friendly welcoming closing In declaring 'Simon **come hither**' this is the Family you belong. And why Unique seen difference is my dorsal fin up. Followed In Open waters- freedom with my swordfish Cousins my fish-sword family.

With & **Without** my Diagnosis the Life Path Number **8** 'Chart', runs true from who my lifelines decided **who Simon** could would turn out be.

Remember I am Simon **With** Asperger's. I am Simon **Without** Asperger's.

This is because through my life I've had the privilege en-living **in both** Spectrum's, (trains of thought).

Yes I have been Simon: (Without A.S/Simon With A.S).

I suspect my truth is **A.S.** never really left **me** it was just... !

I **wasn't aware** (of Simon **With A.S**)....once. Also when I was Simon **Without A.S...** once, I still wasn't aware - yet we presume it was there.

Simply because at Stages **from birth** to **diagnosis** it was invisible naked eye non twigged notice in others seeing my Weirdness yes. Quickly making diagnosis... was 'not' made. Awareness A.S was not once forthcoming.

Fortunately my **C.P.N. Found** I should say thankfully. All the **Classic Symptoms** of **Asperger's** Syndrome in its **Mildest of Forms.** In me.

Now I had a **better excuse** to **explain** my **Weirdness.** That (others) would take a gentler approach now they were informed 'of my new diagnosis'.

Things and things.

Nothing more than following a path of dotted lines, (**someone else** joins up **for you**, not a free reign A.S evolve.

I don't become what others want me become, ((the sheep)). Well that's true. I was a **follower once** look where that got me. Too follow & Lead both will carry nothing ever quite worked out - others are not liking in you.

A Trait of an Asperger's Man. Will always be less inclined to **sheep follow** he rides a Camel of Awkwardness instead cause no one else can Saddle his load just the way his asked excitements lead.

Therefore, his **always left awkward** cause his fighting to keep his alternative plans. The long hard struggles his damned ((yet with a believe he holds)), he pushes through. He sees how right a decision his **hearts eyelid opens**; spectrum heart Vision. Eyes, laying softer blankets (under his Camels Saddling).

I am a Christian under Roman Rule, in my A.S skin (Values worth a Shekel, my Jewish A.S) more so than a Roman Coin of fear, false hope, a dream not a matching **of coins.**

Yet with due respect going out no difference made, is felt.

The mind that is us is filled with information Learning 'we are unable to give a stable love too', a home with an **Open-fire.** A lifted excitement you want we're not from.

Aspergic people no Qualms.

Something to notice Aspergic people are **Aspergic** there's no qualms to this.

An Aspergic grows best when his allowance is growth; into his nice **Asperger** Man.

Putting moulds on him breaks him into who they want him be. He this man/ boy can never completely down his suitcase, in saying! hey **this is where** my Foundations **I build starts.**

Forever sneered at asked too fall in line. With supposed (Normal) so he vetoes our ways.

Uncomfortable in the **Normal Clothes** I am; you are throwing at my feet. Uncomfortable acclimatising in new waters, **told** are the correct **Waters.**

Volunteering Work.

Here is a list I made in suggestions I do.

To say look I am working for my benefit.

Hence making the **taxpayers my** - new employers.

1. **Leaflet Distributor.** (Working for Lib Dems).

2. **Writer** of **Books.** Helping Asperger People like myself. With no hope sell books sold gave in Charity. Raise Money so seen as productive.

3. **Writer** of **Guitar Books.** Theory & Practical. Helps the Learning of Guitar Circulate. Through devoted love, not by law. Show angles of thought orders a Professional man of Music wouldn't have shown 'that's why my books would bring **Fun** to this **Table**'.

4. **Computer Data Input-er.** Helping Job-centres with their paper work on-line. Letters they can forward on, needing large volume circulation distribution for example. Or working for a firm, Job-centre puts me in touch with, to do this similar Job 'if left alone'.

5. **Walking Dogs** & **feeding Cats.** In an old peoples home close by or just in Village help posting my willingness business cards dotted up permissions winked.

6. **Guitar Teacher.** In a radius of the communities, bringing Learning Difficulties on board with me in line with a practical & theoretical aptitude. Worth into their life's. Passing on skills techniques fun excitement purpose, they want to roll out their beds. The free stimulation open them curtains, I'll open doors their learning not compulsory. Special salt watching knowledge. Placed care sensitive to level each Individual progresses. Going over old learning, introducing New Learning. Insuring development. This

training passed on not unhinged.

Coming too me in free will. Signed up to my programme, on ready to Teach. I am of an Intermediate level Guitar myself, no backing my time 'rusted out'.

7. **Useful Guitar Aids.** Making useful carpentry guitar Aids, both for the Acoustic/Electric Guitars, bringing theory & practical applications together in the fore bearing mind of each. Wishing there was an easier way to get through the highways & bi-ways that is Music. Well here I am to the rescue. 'Yet no backing - I rusted'.

8. **A Delivery Drivers job.** From Pizza delivery to delivering your Car parts broken down vehicles in the Country/Motorway Simon's deliverance reaching in time. (This job is conditioned my A.S conditions I must work Alone. Be left alone).

9. **Church Volunteering.** This can be anything from Bell ringing, to sweeping floors, refilling holy water, welcoming guests showing them to their seats. Maintenance fixing broken benches carpentry. Gardening help in the churches yard.

10. **Working** in **Asperger/Autism Homes.** This could mean extend with Organisations free lancing a few hours here & there. Taking people of my orientation out Fishing for the day. Ice skating. Badminton.

Taking **notes** digging at a (Story) my Aspergic Cousins wish to tell. Places I visit homes caring those conditioned on Spectrum's calendar now **including** say their **story.** In with my **books Chapters** dedicate a worthy spot. Future book volumes brought around (we had fun together building). Not a rush hurried thing. Making their life's not just bearable but like they, cannot wait to wake up each day.

Feelings of my hard pushed for time, **in things** I'm better **unfolded.** Such as time on my hands, now dedicate shapes my books to come.

11. **Join an Angling club.** Join an Angling club such as (The Southsea Angling Club in Portsmouth), finding friends at the **Asperger** & **Autism Homes** I work. Asking

them would they help me out to an Interest their showing. An having a ((pint)) once in a while at the bar. Celebrating **I don't know,** a Catch we caught together 4 to 8 lb Cod Plaice, Mackerel.

12. **M.P.** This is quite ambitious maybe an M.P or Representative speaking for those people on my Spectrum without a Voice helping them gain confidence. So they can help me out. Share in life's fortune. Friendship in the high standards. New systems people adapt open. Not forever frightened freedoms too much legislation.

That is more than enough Jobs I briefly shared here with you. I got a lot more. So considerate to my readers family conserving paper space, Ink valuables.

Jobs I have had in times gone by.

1. **Shop fitter/Carpenter & Joiner.**

2. **Making 'Powered Air Brakes'**, for Lorry's, H.G.V.'s, Arctic lorry's.

3. **Domino Pizzas** delivery moped boy.

4. **Perfect Pizza.** Pizza Maker/delivery boy. (Big Yellow Phones on top their Cars. You may remember maybe).

5. **Paper Rounds.** (Tips at Christmas was fun).

6. **Kleeneze.** (Pyramid business stuff, door to door selling.)

7. **Site Work.** Price Work: **working** on my **own** Mortimer in Reading. Whilst working 'part time' as **Bar Man** at the: **Rising Sun Pub.** In Mortimer Reading. Berkshire.

8. **Bar Work.** Other pubs. Friendly atmosphere my A.S can cope.

9. That is enough jobs remembered. Gave in no particular order. Without echoing on just shows jobs paid my Rent. Struggles a survivable living.

10. Jobs I taken on in numbers 10. 11. 12 ever

continued. Is left blank due to pushed for time, saving of rambling paper/ink.

11.

12.

Chapter 11.

My Numerology Life Path Number 8. Simon your, Personal life path number is 8. Number 8.

'What is a Life Path number?'

If ever there was a moment of total transformation Simon, it was the moment of your birth. In that instant, you stepped through a door in time into a new reality -- the reality of human life.

The most important number in your numerology chart is based on the date of your birth, the moment when the curtain goes up in your life.

Even at that moment, you were a person with your own unique character, as unique as your DNA.

Everything that is you existed in potential, much like a play that is about to begin. Your entire life exists as a potential that has been prepared for.

Simon, you have ultimate freedom to do with your life as you like: To fulfil its potential completely, or to make some smaller version of yourself. It all depends upon your effort and commitment.

You make the decisions to fulfil, to whatever extent. The potential life that exists within you.

That is your choice. In this sense, the possible you is implicit during the moment of your birth.

The Life Path number gives us a broad outline of the opportunities, challenges, and lessons we will encounter in this lifetime.

Your Life path is the road you are travelling.

It reveals the opportunities and challenges you will face in life. Your Life Path number is the single most important information available in your Personality Chart!

'What does a life path number of 8 mean'?

Simon, you are gifted with natural leadership and the capacity to accumulate great wealth.

You have great talent for management in all areas of life, especially in business and financial matters. You understand the material world, you intuitively know what makes virtually any enterprise work.

Your talent lies not with the bookkeeping or petty management, but with the greater vision, its purpose, and long range goals.

You are a visionary, and a bit reckless.

You possess the ability to inspire people to join you in your quest, but often they are incapable of seeing what you see.

Therefore, those around you, need your continual guidance, inspiration, and encouragement. You must prod them into action and direct them along the lines of your vision.

You attract financial success more than any other Life Path, but effort is required.

Simon, your challenge in life is to achieve a high degree of detachment, to understand that power and influence must be used for the benefit of mankind.

Those born with the Number 8 Life Path, who do not understand the real and relative value of money are bound to suffer the consequences of greed, they run the risk of losing it all!

You must learn to bounce back from failures and defeats. You have the character and resilience of a true survivor.

It is not uncommon for a person with your Life Path

to experience major reverses, including bankruptcies, financial failure, but you also have the talent and the sheer guts to make more than one fortune, and build many successful enterprises.

More than most people, your failures in marriage can be extremely expensive for you.

Despite the difficulties that life presents, you will experience the satisfaction that comes from material wealth and the power that comes with it.

Business, finance, real estate, law, science (particularly history, archaeology, and physics), publishing, and the management of large institutions.

Are among the vocational fields that suit you best.

You are naturally attracted to positions of influence and leadership, Politics, social work, and teaching are among the many other areas where your abilities can shine.

You are a good judge of character, which aids you well in attracting the right people to you.

Most 8s like large families and sometimes tend to keep others dependent longer than necessary.

Although jovial in nature you are not demonstrative in showing your love and affection.

The desire for luxury and comfort is especially strong in you. Status is very important. You must be careful to avoid living above your means.

Simon, your Life Path treads that dangerous ground where power lies -- and can corrupt.

You may become too self important, arrogant, and domineering, thinking that your way is the only way.

This leads inevitably to isolation and conflict. The people you run the risk of hurting most are those you love, your family and friends.

Be careful of becoming stubborn, intolerant,

overbearing, and impatient.

These characteristics may be born early in the life of an 8 Life Path, who often learn these negative traits, after suffering under a tyrannical parent or a family burdened by repressive religious or intellectual dogmas.

Those with the 8 Life Path usually possess a strong physique, which is a symptom of their inherent strength and resiliency.

Whilst your Life Path number is one of the most important aspects of your numerology profile, there are only 9 main Life Path numbers.

So even though you will no doubt feel a certain resonance with what you read above, it must by its very nature be fairly non-specific.

Written by Hans Decoz.

Simon's personally written 'Life Path Number', was **written by:**

Master Numerologist, **Hans Decoz** himself.

So this is Simon thanking Hans Decoz. x

Hans Decoz, **Hans Asp**erger - was that coincidence?

2 Hans.

Strange 'Aspergic/Autistic notices details so often.'

The Day I was born Chart.

This may Interest you: 'you may say' what is this to do with Asperger's?

Simon has Asperger's so is ((**Day** I was **Born Chart**)) 'connection'.

Since Asperger people, '**like** showing you **who they are**' separate from, their Diagnosis.

Should you believe in the **linking** of **numbers**, Spiritualism, a believe in God/ Jesus, fate destiny, how the 'World was' the **Day I was Born?**

Than you can see: Simon through termed **Non** Aspergeric life, and **with.** A Chart surrounded by events: **18th July 1972,** my date of birth.

And most Importantly you are: (separating the connections found In Asperger Simon) 'in showing him you care' as Simon can disconnect **his** Asperger's.

Once he was thought to be ((**Neuro Typical**)), and 'thinks he is, since told (he is) for so long.'

Simon is just **glad** ((his has Asperger's)).

The reasons diagnosed in him, make it easier, understanding **'on him'.**

He no longer has to conform to the **Neuro typicals ways.**

Why? Well because **Simon's not Neurotypical.**

He **suffers badly** with 'Asperger's' the **Mild Asperger's** representing him.

Here's the **Chart then:**

What was happening in the World, **when Simon was Born** Follows next.

The Day you were Born.

Simon Newell, Born **Tuesday 18th July 1972.**

You are **9861** days young on your **1999 Birthday.**

You were most likely **conceived** on **26th October 1971.**

Biography.

Simon means: **Obedient.**

Birth Day Tuesday: **The God of War.**

July means: **Soft haired.**

Star Sign: **Cancer, Crab - Caring.**

Chinese Year: **Rat - Ambitious Honest, Prone to Spend.**

Birth Stone: Ruby (Contented Mind).

Flower: Lily of the Valley.

Colour: Silver.

Planet: Moon - Intuition. Emotional.

Lucky Numbers: 2 19 30 38 42 45.

Who Shares your Birthday? Richard Branson. Vin Diesel. Audrey Landers.

Sensual Characteristics: You need Romance & Poetry, it can be a real turn on. You are in Love with Love.

And have lots of Mental & Sexual power & energy.

World News: Fighting in devastated North Vietnamese Quang Tri is bitter.

Queens Cousin, William killed in plane crash.

Iceland: Bobby Fischer arrives for Chess Match against Boris Spassky.

Lee Trevino: Wins British Open.

Simon Newell **is Born.**

Medical advances: First Kidney & pancreatic transplant.

Invention: Electric Pocket Calculator.

Reigning Monarch: Queen Elizabeth II.

U.S President: Richard Nixon.

Latest Royal Birth: Nicholas, Son of Duke of Kent.

Prime Minister: Edward Heath.

Opposition Leader: Harold Wilson.

July 1972 Cost of Living. Year 1972 compared to 1999.

	1972	**1999**
Pint of Beer	18p	£1.70
Loaf of Bread	11p	55p
Pound of Butter	22p	£1.58
Newspaper	6p	45p
3 Bedroom House	£9,680	£58,500
Average Car	£1,421	£12,600
Inflation rate	9.1%	3.7%
Yearly Wage	£2,160	£13,400
Gallon of Petrol	37p	£3.40p
20 Cigarettes	30p	£2.80p
Dollar to Pound	2.4	1.67

July 1972 Entertainment.

Most Popular Film: The God Father.

Most Popular Band: Deep Purple.

Most Popular Singer: Don McLean.

Most Popular Song: Puppy Love.

Most Popular Musical: Grease.

Most Popular Trend: Jeans.

Female Oscar Winner: Liza Minnelli.

Male Oscar Winner: Marlon Brando.

U.K BABIES BORN: Boys 414262. Girls 389728.

NOBEL PRIZE WINNER: Heinrich Boll, Language Baby talk.

World Population of those who reached 100 years is:

40,000.

Sport: Grand National Winner: Well to do.

Golf British Open: Lee Trevino.

Cricket Winners: Warwickshire.

Rugby Winners: Gloucestershire.

Wimbledon Winners: Mens: Stan Smith.

Ladies: Billie Jean King.

FA CUP: Leeds Utd 1. Arsenal 0.

Heavyweight Boxing Champ: Joe Frazier.

World Snooker Champion: Alex Higgins.

Here is a Reading I was given by a Clairvoyant.

In an Indoor Shopping Market, at the Tricorn Centre. (before it was pulled down).

It was sort of opposite The One Legged Jockey, clothes shop. Upstairs in 'Charlotte's Superstores', you may Remember, as a Resident of Portsmouth.

I'm not sure of 'year' this Reading came about. Point is, it's one I kept.

She was really good she only charged me £2 to £4's at the time.

This Reading was one of Best Readings given me, serving as how I silhouette myself timetabling.

So here's Simon's Reading many moons ago.

Clairvoyance Reading.

A Stage of nothing happening around your at Prism.

Ending of a Relationship (Past) you have given up on this, which is a good thing.

A New Skill, New Learning situation, Working in a Group

of others, (Positive Stage).

Some sort of acclaim & recognition will come to you.

Higher Education, at a later date, technical skills that will bring you much money.

But beware of attracting Hangers on, People who use you.

Star sign. Cancer.

HERMIT: On a lonely Journey, trying to find more information, in order to survive. Why should I carry on as he is?

Out in a Wilderness no real Growth, Nothing is Comfortable.

Trying to find an Answer, to the Environment he finds in is Hostile.

He is Hiding his face, for some sort reason.

Is Weary of it All.

This is you Simon.

You need to Change, this knowledge, Information, Education.

Hierophant: Hiding his skills Talents.

Powerful Person but is hidden away.

This is you Simon.

Education, Communications, Media, Drama, Theatre, Journalism.

World Togetherness at One with yourself, this is what you want.

Queen of Wands.

Achieve, Successor, Skilled person.

Powerful Enterprising, resourceful Individual.

This is what you want: The Balanced Scales.

Chapter 12.

Guitar Life, Profession or Hobby. Carpentry Projects tied in with Guitar.

Labour my Government choice. Led the way along while reaching my higher Guitar status days. Learning methods techniques over 10yr stretch inbuilt of my time locked in shuttered away my happy World Curtains Open. Scuttled my better tapped autistic capabilities entertaining family and friends a free job where the word economics wasn't my missing '5th A string'.

Where people felt human. I was free of stigmas like Mental health and Politics. They only once were barely buzzwords flicking Oxford Dictionary sound bite meanings of fun non required clarities. Signed off from 'Work' for Life. Diagnosed with A.S. the doctors allowed my progression 'projects' I surrounded lived walked my health feeding the Swans. My adapted life settled happy Alone free movement seized after 2010 new structures.

My academic achievements, home-grown learning was now saddled be folded up neatly in my Chisel bag, laced tied tightly, throw out on your way past the 'Tip bins'.

((We are shrugged off)), to any already built up hard educations alternative thinking man of our Alternative thinking worked his contribution. I stacked my **loyalty card.**

A.S comparisons of, a Spoiled child who had most things as a younger man adapts preference skint/financially stable... spoils you grant potato sacked man's threads (equality) lined velvet inner sleeves. All are welcome at this dinner table.

Bowled over one way thinking, you just agree with messages of, ((It's **the same** for **everyone**)) because!

Favours not looking silly - fitting In. Amasses friends In golden gates. Walking past your own first principles I find upsetting. Disingenuous though understand it is not you at fault for I tagged with you distancing my first Corner healthier stabilities.

This demonstration of power is my **Left Sock** pulled up ((a thumbs up to Alternative thinkers)). With a Right footed Sock falling down that is be-trenched not wrong - nor autistic right.

Or it's **Right Sock** up, left Sock down favouring Right ideology. This means then that **where one** is **favoured** ((one goes under, drops less elastic)). Never is there a balance. Pull both Socks Up on both legs, **now stay up, both socks.** No accepting - meant no equal harmony 100% **cotton.** I see no compromise made.

Someone shall forever lose out a sacrifice made of us the Alternatives in thought. A.S in Thought leaves red oxide rust my doors fall off rubber **tyres.**

Education/Support. Labour Party helped Simon. 10yrs his struggles 'become as good as he became.' We are lucky we have a Labour party who Care.

Promise I showed 'with the taxpayers money' panned out (wasn't hidden). Gave same levels of support (money) as you would pay, any Musician **too perform,** at a **'Concert'.**

Playing the Flute all day (7 days a week unemployed) means you're dedicated not lazy. Worked alternative, your time swings no other valuation more important obsessed different A.S.

You cannot uproot concentrated orange squash with extra Water. Cause 'Employments' calling you, your dedication tastes watery mastering 2 objectives. And why I A.S Master One obsession. Concentration strong.

Sure this World asks you only Work in Employment dedications. Yet what of the earnest man. His mastery his greater influence his (first subject) slices less than a hobby. Is this democracy at work? metal coins spreading abstruse equality. Wrongful angles - I sit rejoiced.

Money out the Public's pocket which ever angle of thought you cage Justice in, is wrongful. Too much Privatizing is OK. Yet my Public mastery besets me I gold Public persuasions. With usage ragtime's effort.

Same as mothers mothering ((doesn't want)) her child going too school, mix with other kids. She mother herself, can **teach** her own **child.** Skills this child bestows open ears. His Job worthy when, coming of age knocks saving the taxpayer in other lights school fees not requiring. Winning hearts & minds.

Textbooks stationary school uniforms, government parents fork-out your curriculum guideline followed. Mother provides better environment, better planned money enthused at work. Wisdom she's entrusted.

It's like some pay with cash. Some will pay via debit card Jeeves old boy, (so really it is this subtle difference), which we talk about. 'Both though are achieving'.

So biased is a 'Monetary system' set loose enjoying life's majestic, non accepting then receptive. African White Russian Indian American so forth and so on all of us everybody not having too be-careful a tip toe friendship my passport keeps walking. One nod of the head stand up sit down 'keep moving'.

Happily accepting Volumes in size with small groups spurring off shake hands reform educate with your World. Only one mindset is today's majority. Tomorrow I walk both Socks Up.

Asperger's ((is my currency - higher functioning)).

Labour Party 1st Care. **Health** comes 1st for others. Over given a choice before we care about economics ((winning through)). So I do Vote Labour.

The **weak man,** is easily manipulated to accept everything as Gospel.

Built communities where 'contributing people' take no Taxes from, those working in Capitalist Society. Works better in my A.S logic. Works without money - effort man's new bit-coin Trading. Trade of Goods. Materials all free. Priced with his **effort**, 'is payment enough'. Man's back and fourth sweat of Traditional.

'Trading left with - those people, who did emulate promise.'

Working with **'what we are'** not deflating us your spare wheel, our promising Roads. Are shared with you as a Cottage we both retreated a woods surrender.

So taxpaying/money is was always well spent, **key ingredient** too paying **Tax.** Those who do **'put In'**, ((cherish fellow humans all creeds)). Educations shown as diverse systems at work, creates excitement.

Without my once 10 year education gift, **gifted.** To us once the **stranger** of **thinkers** In Labour. Meant lining up - in an orderly cue. Handing back like an Army kit. (A Gift I shaped of my prudence) little use to them whom we talk of. Red tape issue - of hit hard addressed.

((My **gift** of Labour Education)) handed back like an old computer you cannot wipe the memory and just forget pleased.

I took control responsibility, over how I spread my benefit received ((my taxpayers money)). Spread pockets education worth the turned around help.

I benefited wisdom sharing knowledge, results man kinds, **lifted spirited** further stage. Require transcending...! thought moulded to my A.S skin, we are pushers of freedom **'giving'** same results. Any Normal person says is right for him. Way he'll work things out... a process thought working 'for him'.

My benefits - is my good faith, courthouse my own mind. Is no different than Governments may do with 'accumulated tax', way **Councils** are handed a life line over their own future. Accumulated tax fish diving from **government** to **Council pots.**

Keeping **my Head down**, getting on with Educations I swim. Not wasting **my time** 'Questions you ask me', slows me.

Furthering myself up high peeks is my Tree Tops. (Stunted blows), tedious filling in of more paperwork **you ask** from me.

Wasted paper, piling my untidy draws.

Tax doesn't have to be Taxing. I beg to differ. You kid-din.

Fun paying Taxes stands a chance of making better decisions. Hearts minds of all blossom in your fairer World. Is a **direction** I'm taken In. And never am I deterred to not follow strong feelings, I wade my boat through. I am tired of a Journey I'll forever follow, 'with few results'. Matters not I am here. I stay.

I breathe easily & freely cause I'm told! Love how we pay In life 'is seen differently by many', through man's existence on Earth.

Had I become ((The good Working Citizen)), who pays his taxes. Paid **taxes** through an array of jobs I had - was paid.

I would as of consequence missed out in a **Self Education** which needs the constant **Concentration** of '**not**', having a **job.** Too ones you're happily prescribing.

Therefore, 'not able' (pay in) taxes myself way you'd like (an all fit in suitable same).

No **movement** no **room** for our Musician friends. Persons requiring a freelance lifestyle. Fore hours demanded of their physical body physical mind, **shows you, tells you,** hours are worth more, great results are achieved of them hours.

The only **negative** as you know by now is, we cannot be both a Working class person who pays Tax, and a Freelance who spends his and her hours practising Ballet dancing, Musicianship. There In **not paying tax.**

Requiring **they/I** ((pay in a Tax)) **I can't.** All this effectively does is ('**split my time**'), with **Work** and balancing becoming Master Musician, in a third arm grown, '**is overloading** a **concentration**'. When really dedication requires you give energy (**to one** or the **other**), never can you accurately be a giver Inside both disciplines.

Quick Sarcasms, say then! 'you know what do then!' 'Stop being this Musician' and get a Job, easily rolled off tongue.

Yet how much good shall be bagged wasted? New corrected good shaping our World. Tortoiseshell inwards our retreat creative input.

In 'performing' for him/her, is us letting them into the free Shows. Energy's I require my performance levels, **not** be **disturbed** dogmas simple man earnest. Left discharged takes less friends, less reward optioned happy - loneliness I took.

All profits I make gives to Charity. Wheels of good hope prosper **my A.S. Help**, work with me/us with Asperger's set your dials GMT in sync.

Oh no not more 'obsessive' A.S. talk. I'll be brief.

You have taken this path such as I (Simon) it is **thought** you will be the **people whom work hardest.** Prove the puddings raising. Ideology I muster too clinging mast of boat.

I'm an alternative **other.** I pay my taxes, back In conundrums given in giving efforts. Same colour **effort gave** I used 'they used', the taxpayer.

Earning money/financial gain pays out on tax expenses, with no special privileges. That common message of ((It is the same for everyone)) rhetorical played record dead spirit accepted talk. So better Taxes too come, actually encourages a tired goat yawning only.

So tell me, when I say it 'like this' to you. Showing you how I see **A.S. Difference suit,** difference between a **Non Taxpaying friend**, scale slide with **Taxpaying** Varieties?

We are **both** ((**working** for a **better World**)), loves a test of humanism. Not about fairness for One person, One group larger only. All people rejoice pay equal tax equal responsibly across the board shown money or shown effort. Combinations of both you chose your choice. Juggled negotiation. Improvement shapes turning, your keys.

A torch not about to lose dimness is A.S strength. The lines I'm guided then draw upon, powerful enterprising, dropped guards let your friends in, 'upping sticks up guard', now friends within stand tall shoulder smart shoulders.

Looking out all compass wheel directions, 'ready battled', light earthed conversations, we negotiate a plan forward circle this compass protect. Isolated demand is your expansion tread eggshells tread water way Asperger prepares.

Show who you **are.** How you contribute in this your World. Thanking you however **small/large** contributions **'you work In'**, it matters not privileges as per fore-mentioned are wiped down as (denied). Your way we are looking for; lift **overriding** factors **here.** Ask nothing more of you, than try a best, we won't knock you - confident.

Our accelerations care to **not tell you** you're **wrong.** 'Happiness we see evidence in' even if you're only one agrees with yourself. Is alright by me our Kid.

Oh but Tax must be paid to pay '**Services - you use**'.

Well then **Special Cards** for the **A.S.** should now be rendered pushed in place deliberately, so **all Services** are **free** with **him,** much like my dental care NHS is free and seeing the G.P.

I/we as an **A.S. Body** of **persons** collective have earned our free tickets, supplied a World we know generously helping out, **our free** con-formative ways offered, often **denied.**

Practically here in says: 'Services' provided each individual (he is gifted, dependent on **offerings**) his proposed, 'he draws up with his World', argues out reasoning.

Depending on **ones** 'ability disability, self reliance.'

Jesus died on the **Cross** for **us,** we all pay in varying ways, Taxpayers/Non Taxpayers, matters not.

A pair of Jeans is just a pair of Jeans, no matter **Designer Labels** (since all help out), everyone is actively seen to work **no matter** murky political dogmas.

No devious ways or tailor me slack what I consider an honest way, 'his mind has told you he works like this', that's tax enough.

Harbouring his A.S. energy '**for** the **Tax**'... you instead take out A.S. minds composite (different in Nature too you). Understanding, replace something with taken.

All ready, fast now **disagrees** with him (him who is respectively different). He is still producing the goods you asked for. As (an **A.S.**) non or less conformist, **everyone** must make sacrifices, less one sided. Two Socks pulled Up.

Why should one person pay taxes, another shouldn't? because the **one** that **didn't** pay **taxes** is one whose had work harder **show his game** 'produces fruit'.

Money the **non** - taxpayer '**made**' he gave to Charity. Even while moaning of unfairness was going on by others. He kept on going.

Jesus kicked down the **market stools,** because of corruption going on around him, money/shekels thrown up in Air slow motion feeling. Giving way too **those** who worked freely.

((**Those**)) could not... pay taxes, their only crime, 'caring' leads to poorness weakness.

Deemed his correct way, is our correct way, seen (by many & few), **he** had **declared** he was **working** freely.

Declaration he's Free of mind declares! is much like taxpayers declares their earnings. Therefore is **Equal** of **payment** when questioned usage promises platitude (what **good** it's **doing**) hard efforts bended or defended. I run exercised along Southsea 'Seafront.'

Jesus is a fair God yes. I am sure money kicked over,

by those who had paid their taxes, was collected say by a simple boy after, '**given back** to **his** people.' (**Distributed** another way again).

Jesus was angry a once thrown to the ground disturbed Market.

Jesus had too **stop** make a point upon **his** people.

Those who could not see wrong doing, 'they thought was right.'

Paying In good taxes still were corrupted, for those **spinners** of **money** collecting, brasher white suits harvested 'Law'.

Not caring for those who paid like, citizen Good Smith unless systematic with Work-abilities is caring. Those not paying our triers dignity.

Grateful you grow in your fairer Society A.S.

Draw closer to **God; Jesus.** Not closer to man with or without Religion. Logical thinker, Religious thinker, matters not no more. I am a Christian.

Test we underwent makes you one thing other, or other thing. Deciding the person you grew.

One day our differences, all seen. Cauldrons **of thought** if good fighting **results**, hands help.

Volunteering e.t.c.

Helping out by Volunteering, a freedom, I am best conditioned. I'm not trying wriggle out of 'Work', I just reiterate forever I require (Work Alone).

My hands, arms, legs, body, head all work ongoing OK. I am best in sync with pressure I know. Any loss of sensation I know, cramps, my own self! is with a numbness 'awkward' best described is! as a lack of Enthusiasm not laziness. I can Work under pressure do all the things I could do when at ease yet, I feel I am running backwards skipping my rope with 'no lift'. Sensations, holding me positions a position, foundations strong roots, built of another's (Interest), the rest of my Working Age! Isn't there holding me keen.

Working any other way is painful against my own pulling chains, though you're correct, I fight through. Fore how else under pressure would I Write a Book. Is a stress Worked my way. And one I can deal with Smiling.

My 'Back' is my worst disability made worse with stress/pressure. I cannot accurately Work this way under mandatory rule of say a Job-centre. I can yes Work under stress pressure so I am not, staunching you what I prefer not do. I just point out my handicaps disadvantages... boot laces less sensation.

Don't misinterpret me 'what I can and cannot do'. I am a fighter I can do all things yet to what form of humanistic, do you see my body pained a Normal

way? I am A.S I have conditions tailoring my excitement keeping moral. I am under a spotlight with discomfort, refused my first conditionings.

I am cramped with numbness, while I Smile pleasing you, carrying your own tasks out.

I don't talk of my painfulness cause it is evident I Work fine in your company. Yet I am losing more friends upsetting an apple cart... I don't bite from.

Energy that is openly, me running through my hearts hands; my Interests wronged is slammed. Painful signalling, my head messages. Messages of stubborn my hands don't flow. Blood mine I am. Then they look Up and see me, saying! he's alright 'see' there is nothing wrong with him. And I Smile again proving their message right.

Enthusiasm I Smile next sings, Normal. How long shall I last pretence cramping my Enthusiasm of their shrivel.

Trying to get out of Work, I'd join the cue of dishonesty... and say my ('Back') is snapped useless. Nevertheless, I know my 'Back' is with unknown pain and Good days. If was work shy! I'd tell you I can't Walk. I'd tell you I can't use my Hands heart and stealth. However this is not my case. I fight through all pains and niggles for I am a fighter too (do-Well).

I can play Guitar I can use my Carpentry tools thy well, so ducking Work isn't my driving force. I want too Work with conditions I hormone fast response, ready portfolio draw an Action Plan up with you Today. Where I am best suited 'my affect results'.

I am Vulnerable easily led, agree 'your way' Often.
I laugh along joke with you knowing your way - is me keeping you pleased, waiting for the collapse. I see no one feathering me 'same energy' because my financial currency isn't one you convert. Your friendship is built on your upper hand strengthening. Normalized a backing you win. Sadly I urge you your correct.

My hands my minding. Looks away, with no sensation no care, any Interest fell short; my Obsession. I run rendering no mandatory compulsion fascinated insecure.

Good to find also a few N.T.s sharing A.S symptoms. What form of diagnosed Normal do you abstain? All like for like closeness diagnosed Mild Asperger's I find I am! A mixed race of A.S and N.T.

Being Asperger's I tend to use my Words interchangeably. I flow a Pen of Normal. Turning Aspergeric Scribbles the next. Running Normal I do so to please a Majority World. Finding home languages my happiest emotions born of A.S. I often tie the wrong rope around the wrong tree. And still call it Home.

Asperger's people want to Work, without control. We ask is this, this wrong?

I whistle along strokes of my Carpenter's Plane, rhythm. Shavings I declare you fair usage, yet how Lawful must we be forever watched.

Shunned then shunted for not producing good Works any other way, then via Normal. My hands operate best A.S. only one way In. That's where my friends live.

My panic attacks are not serious, nor is my o.c.d, lessened when with Authoritative blessings lessening Mental illness, upon a once fit versatile man, bears me better concurrence.

Again, I am not boarding a defence of panic attacks so I may duck (Work), I am Smiling what is denied in me a path I hammer out indentation. With no clarity my dents keep denting crying my Apology. While you rage 'get out', extra over time incurring smoothing a business! of never settled dents.

I guess you could say everyone panics. So is no different than an N.T seeking Yoga Meditation installing calm polarity. A.S and N.T.s share this trait of life.

My panic attacks were mainly due to giving up smoking. And having too Move home 7 to 8 times. With 7 to 8 lots of bad Neighbours who constantly felt it the Norm to Slam Slam their Doors. Cupboards very loudly.

I now Live in a quieter place stopped smoking few years ago the stop start I was before. My panic attacks virtually quickly left me. I now live in a friendlier quieter place nice welcoming neighbours.

Writing Books; Typing. All things following my Instructive mind carried out, makes me of physically sound, well adjusted. Focused on my goals.

Backaches, Stress on my lower back, pulls after any exercising of medium to long range short/long cycle rides out Walking. Pulling lower back, like carrying a 10kg, weight tied dangling.

Especially where I currently live. Surrey Hills. Surrey hills is one word, 'Hilly'.

Moving Home each time because of my previous bad Neighbour's my 'Back' always in such events suffers next followed couple of days. As does Working prolonged time lengths. Is a long list of ((whys)), I keep inviting a (Voluntary plan) forward talked in Job Centre Interviews attended. Full Employment is their better Plan, for me. Although, Full-Time building Up to - in their favour and defence is, something I noticed of recent 'they Care'. And so any form Full Time Work worked with Flexibility, and more Importantly Work Alone. (Is my Workable).

Working Up to 16hours a week later On is where a good start begins for me.

Self-employment another.

When Stationary long periods of Time or Working supple exercised light/hard, my 'Back' is ministered with enough strength I walk cycle Normal carrying pain 2kg weighted Smiled Normality pain resides.

Moving suddenly quickly laying in Bed, I bum shuffle at times periodically my 'Back' with no rhythm negotiating each position 'my Back' with No logic sings heavy with combined perfections great. Each passed month, watches like a Weather Forecast.

Walking around means I must agile in my thinking when Walking, raising posture upright conscience stays of bending correct. I can't zoom off. I plan all thoughts.

My hands empathy no longer loses sensation no longer numbs of dead end feelings Jobs not of my choosing... now my life has moved on following my Instructive mind good attitude and people of decent enlisted angles.

Neighbours currently are worthy of calling helpful playful atmosphere. Ease grand healing of most ills.

My Chakra's alignment.. Head, back, arms hands legs, feet body are out of kilter alignment. I entrust absent healing.

My Coordination is a Chakra of A.S. Along with bad habits hard lessons spicing me out of Sync. I work hard bringing a knitted me forever back; coordinating my Triangles harder than most. Too which some flare their Nostrils as a candid flair of, Mother Natures first ease.

Paying into Society. Earning my independents away from all I distrust is best rooted, entrepreneurial or freelance.

Writing Books I inject 10hours to 14 hours per day. So in this sense my man hours In me increases. With a good steady heart in watchful I am the tiller steering my own ships wheel. Firm hand, gentle.

I find it a shame Autistic people are rarely permitted a **golden ticket** let alone silver permits of use.

I run like a steam locomotive, yet no tapestry of me is a connection of wheels building up pace, nor no horn blowing.

With all my problems it shadows. No full-time Employer, Inspired. He'll require a man he'd better promote with more dollar in the pound his interviewees lining up.

People of my humanity conclude Voluntary Work Ointments Ailments of Special conditions. My pitfalls Worked in. The Voluntary Sector, conducts a Spirit of mine bringing out my best! when things go wrong Autistic to my World. I am losing (Full-time Jobs), Time/energy along with every ones patience. So Working Alone is emphasised.

In peoples 'life', you can have your wanted power, use your **own thoughts,** if your heart is rewarding justly. Whilst God is keeping a close eye on all you do.

My thoughts, judged by Jesus, he judges fairly. I gave **my outstretched arm** said help. Please help.

Help people relax. Create calmness, our educated professors, doctors require a performance level **told** their beloved. Education better learned free way exposed. Not World where learning so much while also fighting an evil World ((whilst **trying** too **do-Well**)), must shall rule out the game.

All you understood, was hex, each man and woman - Policies unto himself. Isn't there a (Match button) fast track uncertainty 'I Agree buttons' 'Disagree'? Terms and conditions on A.S/N.T Conditioned.

Oh no he's asking or telling again.

In this **United World,** it '**don't mean**' you must be (United), yet does mean we are all United in this **realization!** ((**of not** having to **Unite**)). 'So strangely or not this, **Unites us**'.

One Vote, over a 'lesser **people**', don't give you strength too kick out. Denounce another. The person said... **Said look people** I am **with-you** just, **different.** Not joining you as a body of members on all your policy's. Just cause I signed up say too your team, I joined. Or forced join cause I was out Voted. (**Voting systems** that keeps **changing**), is not what Autistic people do.

When you can walk freely put down your aching arms, **say look!** ((I am a Non Changing Person). I'm Changing Person in the World... with so On.

Or! I am **less** agreed with, or I'm more agreed with.

It's only then I believe my personal, you can say we are '**United**', in this way.

Untie your World. Work freely for each others, Trade.

Not satisfied:

You want Work in a World, you're **use too!** ((where money helps the World go around)). It is **all you know...** so you surrender too. Without no more thought. Behavioural patterns you were told were right. Upholding your status, since from the early ages you were told this be the **Norm.** Actually believe so.

Then **split** a World you belong United **into** ((**2 Society's**)).

Find which Society, **produces** the **most** loving high production **seen energies.** Real happy glowing faces real folk. No jealousy for your fellow man.

Is Happiness Goodness, traditional healthy 'clean people', **your goal.** Yes/No?

There is No... (It is Not as Simple as that in my, World A.S).

More about that damn Guitar.

Too give up my Guitar. **I am** surrounded reminded (by the Carpentry), 'made in association Guitar'.

You cannot just all sudden turn the Guitar tap off. Disconnect, discard an Interest. You decided have an **Obsessive Interest In.** No matter **economic** dogma. **An A.S free mind** is apart of your **gifting** offered.

It could essential quite as easily have been **another Subject.** I was throwing all my keen energies at.

What hurts more with fairness Tools allowed usage once, my free thinking mind '**Musician I set Growth**'. Collecting straw feathering a Nest. Month by month, year on year. Making life for myself of Guitar.

The Educational Packages coming along, the **D.V.D.'s** I bought up totalling **£8,000** pounds built library too Educate myself, **no one** on my 'Back' environments I ting a Triangle of once Concentrations.

I am concentrated in this way. Noted for Autistic surrendering. I'm heightening more extra disciplines myself extensive scales, **levels hard maintain** (when not subjected a believe/backing). Along with broken governance analysing scrutiny I'm fighting this, whilst fighting stay strong education I follow. (**I am followed In**).

I cannot just abandon the Focus that is me. My River won't turn back. My soul won't allow me steer an alternative course. This is because I have already laid down 10 years of Ground work **works damn hard.** Meaning I am not about to Pawn my Ring in (the poor price), my sentimental **one man's treasure Gift**). Little **use, left** with **another.** Pawned without Instructions. Comes without Instructions.

The Inner Voice my inner mind **I am sold out** even my hallmarked **mind,** sold out ring ((loses value)). This bears true since no other holds the capacities I work, can see.

I can teach you what I know. **I cannot** teach you to be **me.** (Nor would you wish), you are looking for your own Identity. So I said that's **great.**

You see my 'ring' is custom made. Only I keep documented blueprints (how might I Teach) when **my work,** the **tools I use,** forever, is pawned as not economically viable. Yet economically helpful educated Professors language sustainable.

I gave Signals of an **A.S. back off** warning my cats hiss silenced, my mental health declining.

Signed off for life I once met conditional aptitude cause I cannot inter-react with people on long scale time frames due to my diagnosis my Interests set placements.

Especially those not adapt for Political cares you shouldn't weaken he resolves. It is like asking you too change Character, not Politically winked.

At what point can you not turn an Alternative thinkers mind into 'money'. Raising him a 'tax' he pays you. He wasn't born an Airline Pilot. He wishes not a same following.

There was a 'time' I wasn't made visit a Job Centre every 3 Months because they knew without questioning. **I'm not someone** trusted in a Job **of** the **described manners**. As fell In. Once every 3 years was my expected once Invitation.

Fore my past Medical Examinations many held 'already detailed files'. This meant I could do no more. Mind I am followed. And would Work an agreement Voluntary or otherwise! had such freedoms let me open as I ask I unfold.

I understand the government what they do. Is not a making of their own fault. It is their job to chase up where they can save money. Doing right by our taxpayer. Yet changing my heart **b.p.m** this way, slows tax 'I can pay'.

I open my hand Out - explain look don't you See, I work this Way. Why can you not Work with my Offerings I come tailored. Of Course Job Centres are 100% better these Days. A lot of my experience I talk of is of an Older Day Welfare born after Labour lost power. I am not Conservative minded at all as you know. Though in defence of a party that isn't who I am. Let me say they have kept Improving and therefore (I am finding Help) in Today's struggling World.

Earn & **pay** from the Natural source keeps my long Interests Encouraged.

Open heart Natural flow (**my only** asked **Condition**). Swim currents helping out, In Churches sweeping floors. Making my life the joy I seek. This is how my hearing works. Without a broken heart, a broken formation crippled no care just pay damn you. No Incentive.

A **half Inch** thick **booklet** they'd have me fill in with questions you had to ((commit to an answer, 1 2 3 or 4)), **with none** of the **Answers**, representing me in **any no shape way.** Obligations of strict & hardy Authoritarian backbone crushes.

I have a Guitar tattoo 'on right - my upper arm', which when I show others, others see my tattoo, cause it is a hot day. So on display.

They say Simon your tattoo, is '**upside down**', which to them it must seem as so; viewed looking at me the Stranger perplexed.

In this World I view my Guitar tattoo, seen 'right way up'. So does **persons** looking over my shoulder seen gravity correct.

My Guitar tattoo has become apart of who I am. I did not know I would have an Obsession with Guitar Theory at young ages. In later life. It just sort of happened **like this,** lament spoke.

It is just a hobby I choose '**stuck** too'.

It is the One thing apart from Carpentry. I was trying Master, **if you like.**

I had too walk away from my learning studies after having almost no problems in learning Guitar of 8yr/14yr period amassing; tools mind I engineered mind **loyalty.**

The Day (a **Guitarist Union**) **is formed** to say look dedicating all your energy too guitar because this is the **blood sweat** & **tears** you do **pouring In.** Advances New Vocational. Recognitions.

Movements for those who spend their Energy as wisely.

So (government Schemes) become Guitar Youth and Adult Clubs. With 'Guitar Workshops' running. A root into employment or simply paying tax in a (Stamp Book) gave of know hows. Funds entertainment our Club 'lays On'.

Meetings bringing in 'honest Revenue' Autistic man Landscapes a Plan.

Acceptable **excuse not** to **Work** formative controls. 'A Club of people come together **better their skills**, play and pay World; freer ways.

Giving up, not giving up.

Given up Guitar now.

(**Secretly** I still Play, **Shush** though). Only a hobby these Days In. Plucking Strings.. finger-style/Plectrum (**active** lessened **willpower**).

Raising of your believes is healthy you asked not **another** follow (just respect), just Listen.

All of my **Carpentry made projects** over the years stay (covered in dust sheets) 'Guitar Aids'. Folded **Inwards on myself**, because (good work seen) produced with productive usage works my mind I gave free Tax. Direct effort. Take it away. Next Project please.

A **Coffee Table** I made cost more than **£800** at the 'time'. (2 years) in the Making. **Guitars fingerboard** built runs through her **middle.** Shows all the Musical **7 Notes. A** through to **G...** then back to **A** in a circle.

All my Hard work '**slid-den** into the **River Thames**', get a Job rings no truth 'Work' I finite no other. Passion my common goals distracting where I run connecting friends, must we all share same friends reaps no rooms no adjustments. Set stone clauses with no amendments. Square dancing a bachelors rhythm.

Fighting out Principles (saves a man time) fore no changing is 'found' in him after held debates remain (no different) not asked 'turn his stems' re-debates.

Try kept a 'high Moral' we not only fight, disagree/ agrees. (We fight ourselves) **much doubt** placed the doubt bags out in us strategically.

Authority we Saluted happy in Traditional Days, 'changed'. Authority once was Special. I miss the Godliness Holy spirit she sang of.

Morality of human thing going on. Special Moments lost, saddens.

You must fight for your believes hope others join you without urging. Accept pictures you 'thought, fought' right & wrongs **stood** stand for **In.** Wishing on a replica match; without persuasion.

Helps you keep a sanity; should you walk in **Minority aloofness.** It matters not you; **didn't** fit **In.**

Asperger's my Autistic releasing - shall **talk** for an **obsessively** long time symptom of many Asperg. Shall consider Hard-work quietly worked away from Lime light; my enjoyment.

So not having live up to performing always **when it is** required **of you,** was another reason I was setting freedom laws in placements like bottled Sands - colours! layer. Childhood your friends collectives.

Already I had left it late in life started learn my Instrument Guitar. At **30ish.** Yet didn't deter me. Obsession.

Battling the Theories of Music later on in life not only battling to be become **No 1,** but to be told being this No 1, is unfair on the taxpayer, **which giving its due it was.**

But what was I to do?

Throwaway a Principality, I was trained in. Home grown manner, cause 'ruling' is tabling a New Supper.

Were they trying to point out to me, something I hadn't known before?

Was I starting to agree with them?

Well it is a Batman Question isn't it. My best **Bat Answer** is!

The answer is Yes. I did feel ashamed of spending my taxpayers money, 'given in education to me', in a **through** eyes **thought.**

I used spent **in Education this** I talk of. Helps, no confident persons' Societies rejection; too which I know I am One.

So you Pinstripe, the **good** & **bad** you see in all Party Elects.

Can't Vote in a Voting system, because... you are a **little bit of all** and none of the Party's. Not laying down a suitcase hand of cards pristine in One Party.

I (don't change) my trials of thought A.S. I hast am strong Inside.

I had a Neighbour.

I have a Neighbour where I once lived his name, **Nathan.** He plays **Acoustic Guitar** also. We one day had a Guitar Jam together he was really good, he could play **Popular Songs.**

And just 'Songs he had made on the fly', from his **own memory.**

He had a bit of Rapper Influence, to him Character of his oiling, which I am not into myself.

It is just not who I am. But this guy Nathan was very good.

He had (his Capo) on at the 5th Fret. (device used in raising or lowering the guitars pitch so you may gravitate **with** your, own **voices pitch**).

And he was playing the Chords:

Am. G. F. E.

I believe it was.

Which is a nice Chord Progression, that I'm found finding fond. 'Sounds works', **good** in all, **situations.**

With a Singing Voice layered on top or underneath, living to your train of thoughts you can make most 'lyrics' written or scribbled down a 'match' with voice harmonizing your Instrument while your Instrument compliments your Singing Voice. Just with simple Chords you come by. You should try it yourself.

We must have **between us** - Sung & played 50 to 70 Songs, that day.

In the space of time the Sun was shining the hottest, bottles of Lemonade by our-side.

Awakening up the Street **in our Music** people stop were stopping by 'chatting or watching', some people just keep on walking **with** a **slowing down in Interest.** Tapping my foot with Nathan's we kept our Rhythm glancing at people in Awe of us. We Smiled at each other bopping; and Jammed - some more.

I didn't intend play 'have a Jam with Nathan', my Neighbour.

I was 'walking by myself', I noticed he had only **5 strings** on his **Guitar.** So I said!

Nathan. I have a spare, **H/E String**, stay here...

I'll go fetch.

I had never met Nathan before this, so this is how our **once off Jam** occurred.

It is a shame I got Asperger's I couldn't have just, stayed friends with Nathan.

I just feel I like helping people. Then moving away.

Just giving the odd hello's here & there. Is more than enough I can handle.

I often think of our Jam. I hope Nathan his doing OK. I must have seemed rude to him **Liking him,** (One minute helping him), 'him helping me' then **wanting** my own **space again.**

My friend Nathan had a **little gypsy** In him. I believe.

So although I liked him with much love on this side of my heart. I took the cautious approach, same as I do with all people, same they'd understandably do with me.

Yes you may say well we all are cautious (but you can't say), more cautious than Asperger Spectrum.

Why? cause we are '**added extra - Caution**' in mixing and then staying friends.

Chapter 13.

Ending of my 2nd book. Strange place to leave an ending Simon.

Do you know what scares me the most writing a book.

Is when I am out in the World strangers I pass, know not, or see an Author. They just see Simon who has Asperger's and they don't even know this.

They just see another good reason get angry cause locked in their world. They believe we cannot see how great they are. These same people, they've **respected themselves** so much whilst (pushing through you), they forgot to share respect we gave them of 'forgiveness'. Looking at us strangely, might be very worthless denouncing, stares upon us. Ready, lowers your body count intentions.

Like they are miming a message to you, that the (Freedom they provide before you) is something we may not rejoice in. 'You must show **unhappy grumpy bear**' as a joins their extended club.

Forever feel; unhappy. I walked away heave-ho out lifts and carries.

Why people get angry - they feel you are not giving them those right doses of respect. They require passing you in successfully. And a Smile or two would not go a miss.

When you do respect them, they think you are looking at them too much. **So never** can you Win.

When an Author, 'you should see in all people'.

Treat, all people as film Stars. For if you are not you're bagging wins so you look good in the pump only.

Too how **each person** 'is in the mood' (his in with you today) as you pass him by, then another; & another; & another; & another; yes lots of **another/others.**

Different people keep passing **us/you by,** on our disciplined paths. We are trying to be **the nice people,** some respecting the nice you emulated, some not. So we give up some days when showing niceness is mixed with... angry & nice people.

I always remember 'the people who smiled' at me.

And who gave me more **pain** too **carry** back **home** with me.

We in our mind, as an A.S., **typical example** such as **me,** can be really getting along swimmingly, we take lots of great smiles good energy given to us, in the given moments, cherished memories, we are surrounding ourselves in with today, tomorrow, next week. That's always, too help us move along.

Individual movements 'of heavy hard always too fight life's people, **seen** as the other **one face'.** Bottomless basket of Apples is the bad energy angry (faces).

Meaning: **good energy happy smiling faces** is Asperger's filling building his basket in apples, holding onto his apples not wishing lose the ripeness. His good energy is in continual building, remembered. To a bad unhappy angry faces, we lose, hard obtained (Goods) easily.

Dropping losing Apples. He already collected along the way. This is the Asperger's **basket emptying.** Starting again & again (this cycle of), collecting confidence, losing it, collect confidence losing it, collecting, apples falling through the holes.

Then of course the **ones who gave us** or snapped us in **another mood,** from the happy happy happy mood, (I & others), 'keep giving too others'. Others give too others. **In turn gave** too **me,** broke me a little, then them I only can suspect. Then what happens is A.S. are rude or go into a meltdown, misunderstand further.

It hurts yes it did...and yes it does. This process 'is a' (circle) **not with**, an **ending conclusion.** In sight any time soon.

When **not all people** are **Smiling, 'all** the **same'**, you're left questioning? (Is there something I'm doing at all wrong as a human being). You start question yourself 'you ask yourself' **why were** some people **not smiling.**

On saying, it is **not easy** to walk past another Smiling, 'me giving the good energy', **then knocked for my/your efforts.** 'You thought you'd be thanked' (I should know right!), I have come across this more than often, - so did you?

It is also hard dare I say when, people 'are Nice' to 'me'. Especially when it's this very asking, **I yielded** the **seeing in you.** Asperger friend asked! - You give.

Too express the **body language** that is **solely me,** 'thee others might expect (I give)', by saying - **Thank you** too! Them/and You back, whom gave! what I have asked for in my books. Scratches your own heads in disbelieve; the **N.T.s** and inclusive ways 'Asperger' uncomfortably thanked you. Thine not intentional, it is painful and comes out sarcastic mostly, always.

We are more than aware of how, **our receivers** find us rude. With equal times when (the awareness in us) **we switch off,** so we could be rude too you our overload. 'And not be aware'. (In both situations). This is how an Asperger's mind copes.

He'll (over-ride) what you expect of him, what you'd expect him to say.

The reason an Asperger hardened his tension like this, **is!** 'As one' **exampled:** he has already (Thanked you countless in his mind). Problem is showing this 'internal inside thank you... I do'. **Is** too **cheesy over thanking yous.** And too heartless too under thank you.

Thanking you Mediocre isn't gutsy either, so best not decreed. This builds us extra awkward for we are always, wrong.

Most times we adopt a heartless approach letting the nay Sayers, disapprove our arrogant ways. Fore it is clear had I bagged kindness disapproval seeps (whilst this is going on). No one realizes our rudeness was with a **silenced voice** that; Thanked you **100 times.**

So what was I to do? Hang around. I behaviour as typical Asperger's. Family I belong.

Look very close around! **N.T.s share** - Trait's of **A.S Rudeness.** These Rudeness's both A.S.s and N.T.s are found doing. Do not resemble each Other. You can divide a poker stick down the middle distinguishing the Make-Up's A.S decree a rudeness born of A.S Scent.

Our Autistic mastery is stronger born **Rudeness** and why I came in diagnosed **Autistic.**

A missing A.S. **Thank-you - tool, 'we'** cannot give you praise. Stillness saddens us heavier than Normals (missing Thank yous). A.S, and Normals leave out. Aren't paralleled same. When Onlookers...long passed.

More pains/awkwardness you see in Asperger's people definitive. A one selection designated spectrum tree house is where we hang out, Smile.

So even though I make efforts looking for Kindness behaviour in others. You yourself shall wonder why you bothered. Yet come 2 minutes down the Road I was **taping your Aura Thanking you.**

Only way Asperger people know how to. 'So Only, so do.'

More tamped Up 'Asperger **are.**'

Had we not (thanked persons') the way you hoped it plan. **Having** Asperger's you would understand why (we cry Inside) - (the thank yous) you do not **see in us.**

The nasty **bad energy givers** who make you feel how much they, disapprove you (even with all the great smiles you gave handed), understanding looks my awkward landings. 'Made me realise' these people had not fair good starts. Or maybe I broke their coolness being too friendly.

Are they **lost** in the **World** without no Immediate Family to **turn too?** Anger subjected 'the genuine who they are' **with no excuse** uncontrollable behaviour. Usually No

Logic brings Logic. Then I see their Awkward behaviour is not A.S it is N.T and I wait with him because I know 'he, - like me' (he don't wish be Understood).

Are they withdrawn into a box **like me?** are they making it in life on their, own Merits.

The unconnected irregular maintained **angry** at **persons** & **people** a selection few people - singles out. 'Personally relieves a little pain pent'. Struggle **he himself** goes through.

Are they? 'young, busy looking damn fine'. Or is my Awkward A.S a different kind of Awkward. N.T standards.

Is this why they 'shed attitude' onto others. They are wanting a fairer easier World also... perhaps built self-centred different to Asperg self centres clumsy. Looking good in with peers is, unknown standing thoughtless Mirrors.

Ones I analyse. **A.S** myself 'asking ourselves', why they are like this '**like us**' before the once? Were they friendly **Awkward.** Autistic noted?

Yet changed themselves as (Survival without smiles), was easier apparently to fit in, shirking the anger is all theirs, **relieved** a bit more **pain lessened,** 'they did have', put on others carry their non savouries.

A love, room permission grow in this **World** was felt to be told indirectly, this is **Weak persons renderings.** And why so many suffer the boyhood tactics, (of... weakness is not allowed). And why Spectrum Calendared shan't Fit In.

We assert ourselves away from inborn manners, cause otherwise rarely **listened too.** Hence looked upon as an easy touch.

I personally find Smiling & Good Energy people work harder. More than. Any other **type of human stereo-type singleton.** I have ever had the best fortune too unfold. A same love respect given, come across.

My philosophy on this angled approach to how we deal

with do you become '**heavy** & **boisterous**', 'angry & non smiling towards people'?

Or 'meek & mild', '**soft** & **courageous**', 'hard but fair', 'strong but soft'?

Had I to be 'angry & non complimentary towards another'. Or just my preferred Nice. Being A.S I find I am not well Received with only 2 echo's.

Both favour no slack the slips of A.S creeping, my brokered self In mixing (Normal Circles), it starts Well, Ends soggy beer mats.

Respected in a peer group pressured way (for this reason only), **under** their rules of **love** I find no solace rubbing approval unless love is loving a state of mind Autistic, I bring myself controlled.

Disregard no man's feelings as is, I do Internal. External me you don't see.

You'll see Asperger people **not fitting In** philosophies of them who, I speak.

Adapted One look mindset. We Asperger walk away.

Too be **loved** by **more people,** just so shown you make the Grade of worsening ill fought thoughts, you strength mustered walked away away away. You are sometimes **led into** '**agree too**' without, asking yourself (if you actually do), when the mask is loosened for you.

In other words you are instead given a choice **too step back, to be yourself.** Through non fear tactics, that it's OK, stick-out like a sore thumb. Secretly 'you feel comfortable about', cause you know what your **right** & **wrong** means to you.

Or you're hoping, you - think do.

Nonsensical following the devil's path, too be in a place 'of others' Worshipping at one another's feet, bent in the leg bowing down (wrong reasoned).

Real love respect 'gives' (Immediate). Not asked for I, believe. Felt when you are not expecting rewards expecting gain - is wrong shoes. Be Shrewd at the ends, for the efforts you pursue, **love** of **given,** before taken.

Or taking nothing at all.

Is when you can pat yourself on your back. Reward self freely.

Then you will swim in Riches Welfares of man's heart, '**C**onjure, **C**ontain, **C**onvert, **C**urrency, **C**orrectly' the **5 C.'s** paste of War Colours battles already won.

The currency of: **L**ife, **L**ove, **L**iberalism, **L**aughter, **L**etting in, the **5 L.'s.**

Non Smile Tax.

Non Smiler - Tax policy '**Tax**' brought about as a Policy since, unfair to ask everyone in World too do a Well in life. Without the Smiles around.

Selected **few handful**, weigh In damaging Work-ability patterns of: Taxpaying man Vulnerable. By not receiving Smiles or at least friendliness of joy a Work-force builds you healthy. Taxpaying men pitch in Strong jumping out of bed without mandatory whips.

His long lasting Job Is - netting you, Tax Security. Is! Vulnerable man Smiling cause his powered a Contribution 'he Gives'. A World at ease his In. Makes sense. Furthermore, sits In your best Interest strength of an OX caring Good people, strong Tax gravitating Willpower tax, growths You.

Helps out, all another others. Healthy, happy sense of Aura, less jealousy running deep. Or 'not Smiling a feel good factor too your other fellow **Man's welcoming**' **I** hadst wrong, let's us (Smile Tax) reasoning.

Bereavement aside mourning and depression is however acceptable thought about.

Seen as more of a ((**Fine** Insensitive)), than an extra Tax penalty paid. (And you **don't have too** Pay It). Your Helps observed noted. The up and down you spreading less Misery onto those trying be your Friend.

Spectra minds can work overtime, thinking up why?, caught on the spurge in the hop, someone else has changed your happy mood.

Given to you by (good others), and so **unravelling** all tied up **good work placed in you.** 'Given too you before hand.'

Every now and again, all Good placed with You, **some people** are **not playing fair,** letting good in you grow messaged, as shouldn't. Allowing **not.** Breaking you, the way they shouldn't.

Rather they feel the need too nip away at you **not just you,** 'others they can make miserable', when really these '**bad - doers**', (are given good placed with them), or same placed good fortune, (you had), or so it's thought, so **why?**

The mind cannot always be forgiving to another, when ((non smiles)), **stinking attitudes** are left with **me,** him and her. 'Too then be', **the thankful.**

Picked up by the affected, though yes we do **find** power **forgive.**

Finding (a use) for them ('**left** with **yous**') without, **good intentions.** I'll now only pop them in my cupboard draw-side, non Smiler label.

All left burdens with us 'quickly forgotten by', who we are calling **him,** or **non compliant.**

For burdens of their burden is all too much A.S brain now instantly simulate. Pre-frontal **brain cortex** by me I Inherit. Including any slow moving adjustments (his had make made again), **set backs** wanting hinder already maximum strides, I move life's Rhythm Autistic.

We pay an equal fairness on what decisions, or drastic action, **I/he** the **A.S. man** (had to give in heats of the moment) someone taunting another for example.

I Thought you know what those who keep the kept Smiling through! (are still damaged by another others). What with instances of say, the **slamming** of **doors.** More

slamming of **doors.** You know who you are by descending.

Purposely follows lead trends, so you feel their same **Misery.**

For being once respectful, quietly spoken, gentle too greater man's needs, disregarded **not allowed** grow. There is no one Solace way too please.

They get jealous when an another others, are **Happy,** 'they want what you got.'

(We said they can have it), 'yet still hurt the **gifts** of **life** - we **fragile gave'.** No searching (what they are), in rewards we find, they should of.

Never not too late, find something, their good at they find. A cleansed heart.

So we growth an honest admiration an honest forgiveness giving honestly instead, cause that is my feelings. No matter how shaken it today.

'Not' made conscious forgiveness's all basking like crocodiles as, we require Pink Flamingos.

No one can tell 'referred thems' I have Aspergic tendencies. (Since people we rely on) know not we are together **at times**, when we are.

Yet **we're together** 'one sided togetherness', hoping a **2 sided togetherness** will be along soon.

So only **'us,** aware we are **Here**', locks no universal togetherness and him thinking, I am a N.T. Normal. Though Weird, he concludes.

So all another Sees, should he be fortunate/unfortunate, **pass me** by in my tracks and his, is! some 'Weir-do', they call a Stranger.

I'm looking right back at him squarely eyes, believing him to be the stranger crossing my path.

So we both want too get **on by,** 'with a little of locking of the horns', like billy goats gruff, horn fighting, declaring their space, independence.

The messages of this fight, continues in an ever going loop, **locking horns**, with a **new strangers**, 'the same fight processes', **we hadst** with our **last passer bys.** This fight passes to another/others, as we go further & further down the road **meeting Smiles** & **Angry people.** At **unknown** rates.

Should you be the unfortunate one, **coming from** the **other inner directions**, climbing upwards in hill slopes, a freedom message of better communications, can & will form. 'In you.'

Cause you know you're at a disadvantage, therefore smile harder. **Those you** pretend you **like.** Just to get on by.

The more you do this, moving & passing through others, (as one exampled), 'freely turns more considered bad people', Over as Good peoples, as **I'm** passing on **'good will'** **not** with **just One.** But all humans I'm, passing.

In the Seen hope worth my while.

Not because it's an effort, cause look it feels right to do.

Sort of communication fought openly hands, gives you back your! once remembered better Sunny World.

You see they 'other people', as I see them I don't care about them, **I don't know them**, so I am guessing they think the same.

Whilst accepting although this is perhaps true depending on levels of kindness shown or not so, should if nothing else, let us be **Civil.**

They don't know I am a Weir-do with reasons attaching me Weird 'the pass me by people'. Reasons why I am your Weir-do with labels A.S.

You do see why I say 'diagnosed Aspergic' should be handed his own **Army chains** around his neck. Aware says! **'look out** this **guy is A.S.**

Same if you were Diabetic so forth... Ambulance Staff, General Public - people, Medics, need quick this information **when** called upon.

When you are exampled A.S who is unconscious, having a meltdown (that you cannot speak communicate) those whose **job recognizes you** with **I.D.** essential. So look if nothing else carry - Bank, debit - credit - cards. Mobile phone (draw quick informations).

Or get Micro-chipped tattooed... do something.

Check for example 'your Blood group' tattooed.

((A Positive)). Whatever this may be.

Quick info slam, **quicker** than yesterday.

Should you be unconscious pulls out - just one!
Why Information taken by appointed medics. Is your responsibility.

Memories flooding back Army memory lane.

I have 'No Empty cases Blank or Live Rounds' live ammunition, Pyrotechnics, in my possession Sir.

This was a declaration made in my Army, after an Exercise ended or Weekend ended. Quickly scrambled away 'we were then dismissed' by our Sergeant Major.

Our Sergeant Major was 'Mr McGowan' brilliant man we called him ((**Dad**)), because he was like a dad. You could rely on him, Rifles back in the Armoury, and yes home we went.

So on this note: I'd like to say with an Army influence running through me, please.

I Always have **No**, 'angry thoughts.' ill intent, conceived ideas, wrongful doings, unhappy faces, or bad or malicious intents towards another to hinder his unfolding, **not** found of in my possession **Sir.**

Salute dignified.

Hopefully you can see the fun an Aspergic member of society has In life? Shares In life. **Fun** rubbed off symptoms emphasis within you. Carry in a glow bag, so not lost.

Maybe just maybe. It is time ask are you **Aspergic.** You or a person you know. Love in symptoms I emulate over.

And if so look how **fantastic.**

Another member jumps on board with us welcome. Our Autistic Family. One of **our own** love not bought.

Chapter 14.

The Word Disability.

Part of the problem with the word 'disabilities', Is that it immediately suggests an inability to: See, Hear, Walk. Or do many large number other things took on granted.

But what of people who cannot feel? Can't talk about their feelings? Manage their feeling ways, constructive?

What of people able form not, close strong relationships?

People who cannot find fulfilment in their life's, those who have lost hope. Who live in disappointment now bitterness. Shadows his kind heart carries far too many famous people clogging his own 'simple needs'. His disability he Cares with a big heart - he went unnoticed - for you.

Finds, found is his own life, receives no joy. His hidden disability of he Cares, he's wrangled no better solution a Character he said he'll help you out. Sacrifice he gave! he stayed poor for you, All. Amen.

These, it seems to me, **are** the **real disabilities.**

These, it seems too me, **are** your **A.S.s / N.T.s** often knocked, our real troopers often those poor people found downtrodden in Soup Kitchens a lost man. Amen.

Fire Hydrant.

An Asperger may undergo, feels like, he has a Fire hydrant fire extinguisher growing inside him, Autistic 'He and She knows' not knows how; they might disperse throwaway. A fire hydrant man's Character, he Walks strangely amongst his Crowd.

Asperger builds tools 'reminding him', fortresses laid down. The big why? he, cannot Change. Everything put up before me, before you, **can't** be **changed** around. He's planted his first bulbs, **set out** in a **certain order.** Once set don't change, our glue isn't that strong. When moved, changed, pulled around Character, of your Character.

So when (you feel) some people (can change, & some cannot), there is differenced reasons layering, mind pattern, where you 1st must 'look', lessen **A.S.'s** aggravate.

Especially a someone who has been 'told to you', **he has** diagnosed **Asperger's** lookout signs, show transparent awkward messaging.

Run a Tap clear understand conditioning figured. Lay communicate better beacons.

A.S is sketched - that falls to diverse arrays, divisions a Label.

With a way found we Calendar Autistic our beacons, mostly locked deadlocks (with, Normal World).

I held something in my hands - sensitive, 'my heart hands'.

Turn work in unison over, shown way a non-believing World works growth, I Autistic believing am, not from.

Instilled in me, is only my sighted vision. I show you.

Let me grow my developed wish. No Spokes.

Fuzzy Hearing. Talk.

A.S. people Autism, others relating Conditions from our Spectrum generally, connecting directly to, Indirectly to. ((**Fuzzy Hearing**)) Is my next Lectured talk.

I/my Asperger counterparts, must accept all we Hear, 'Using Fuzzy Hearing'. What I mean by this is simple, we select, choose, tuning what we want too Hear. Accurately quickly, not the same as N.T. alignments ways when they chose not too hear.

Fuzzing out distorting Noises/unwanted Noise that plagues, rejects fast with people A.S. the Happy cotton wool we use. A necessity aid for our survival. Against light distractions or heavy Noises ready to plague, we react kick out fast. Or we suffer distraction inwards of ourselves, wishing too menace. More so than an N.T can seemingly, joke it off.

Noises, good noises allowed created, Is in an ambiance our Normal river flows at peace, collected noise fuzz. Our hearing baffled soft wire wool.

This may Play out in a range of A.S.'s, on the Spectrum Calender alike.

So after saying so, here's what I mean. An A.S has an old fashioned Tape recorder on spools playing in his mind, (if you will), of all the Good Noises/ Sounds. Centre's his groundings to an Earth terminal safety nets we build for a better future.

We must Hear all things told our way, then '**we** can **accept**' you on your accepts before braving what outsides World terms as (progression In us), a Changing of us, is not advised in my first and last opinions.

The noises & sounds/voices, that play havoc to an Interior wiring of an A.S. How he is wired from birth, rejects noises at bullet speeds, If he's telling you this is harming him. That's not your Signal to carry on, he made you aware like a King cobra warns. In other words, it hurts decentralising trying to destabilise hearing his A.S language, Originates seen diagnosis. Dragging affect, on movements his otherwise uncomfortable language he comes.

Only (happiness hearing sounds) are running through the temples of the A.S.'s peaceful rivers.

It took the Spectrum disorder along time tweak the ever so quiet rivers, (he's running in him) throughout him), to a performance level '**dedicatory** required'.

With good people set in place.

This maintenance of discipline, you better push through with, when the better ways of thinking, high standards of wasting less energy, is put to better use, wise.

Can't pay, cannot afford yet pays effort his progress. Mind they're developing.

Fuzzy Hearing has **Yin** & **Yang** affects, in so much as (it teaches you to hold, truth & happy sounds). Carried even when we, are **lesser people**, represented by A.S.'s.

Scrutinized, shut down immediately, breathing less accepted thoughts.

Because we're not dancing getting drunk in celebrations as, '**soon quick,** to celebrate **people do**'. In one thought channel we tell you straight away what is right or wrong thinking cohering correct us.

The 'Meltdowns' are not a stamping of feet so we may get our own way, it is quite contrary.

Meltdowns are nothing, if anything at all, connected; not having **our burgers evenly cooked**, or we will complain.

However this '**is**' what a Meltdown resembles, contrary to our burgers flipped right. In session A.S.'s have Meltdowns, 1st seen rule in us as the (Yang effect). If it was Yang we born lodgings into, If it was Yang we found no perfect burger whilst benefiting Yang healing.

So here it is:

A Meltdown is when an A.S., such as myself Mild exampling, Autism as the strong examples, have **built up** '**Hearing wave**' patterns perform frequency known, he knows. Frequency loved ones Parents know about. Disturbed asked re-shape, built-up, inherited **programming**, (that is identifying him as him and us as us), is inside furthering representations **me others,** living the Spectrum, 'is tampered quite often non-acceptance', frequency I operate on, 'is our very own **lifeline**'.

You do see why we **stay protective**, keeping our wiring clean tidy takes much dedication, a slight glitch saying don't you dare think like this **sets off** Chimed whistles **set in us,** leaving you with my deadly toxin is not pretty. No fault of our own, Meltdowns in full swing, the ugliness of Asperger's Syndrome.

Pressured 'unfair, our freedom represses' thinkers thoughts are Square one gone back. We lash out the unfolded tail between our legs, snap you one lashing a provoked reaction, we felt perhaps you had coming, one we took no control over.

Don't bash ridicule Spectrum. He's not bowing down (pleasing you). 'Praise him', turn away from him, accept him, love him, debate him, cry him, treat him as though A.S Is also Normal.

Tell him, that's OK Son. I sort of knew this would never be easy, (the **you** & **me thing**). Say, let us be friends opposite coins.

Or Say, 'A novel way to think, **Mr A.S. Man.**'

Say not a problem we'll swing & keep, all Methodical juice creams, **'you** & **we'**, swim in groups thousands safety.

Kept clean by the, **Understands.**

Bigger enough know, smart enough take on board. (You'll never change A.S.'s Zebra-stripes).

Black & White, **Yin** & Yang. 'Meltdowns one side' fixed so strongly, as **Yin** perhaps. Because One side must keep it balanced, with **fair opposite.**

Challenged them! 'you **don't do**', genuine truth at work (in you, how you work). Genuine truth 'how I work', with no thrills added to hinder.

Fair to say, then '**Fuzzy Hearing** & **Meltdowns**' go hand within hand. That where there's a **Meltdown,** there's a **Fuzzing Hearing.** Toxin release follows **Warn**ing **you** he can't change, help how he thinks.

Warnings you best as sweet smiling patient friendly

powers carry him. A.S., stepping up pushing all you carry 'as **enemy**' faraway distance, he/me cave muster between 'the **Us**'.. the **black** & white opposites.

So Summing up '**Fuzzing Hearing**' goes like this:

Fuzzy Hearing a protector inclusion of 'Meltdowns'. Revs at a steady rate 'till deterred ask perform' performance, 'that is another's Identity', making **us not us**, making us, 'you'.

Why this a problem? Well 1stly, said in my 1st Book, **everyone** in **life** looks too

much like the **same**. 2nd, N.T.s spoke generally! they infuse 'they are' these Characters someone, somewhat different; to their other counterpart N.T.s, when A.S., honestly! I do see only a certain One universal Character that they are all, (performed as). Bonding holds of the togetherness they kid themselves, we like too pretend, we are. This is perhaps because it really is easier unchallenged this way.

Even when changing a new Imagery You fashion Today - coming across, there is a label unspoken; that Punks a person belonging Groupings, sectioned as this/that.

There is no difference in people from one to next everyone stereotypes in a One certain Band. Or rather cause people stay controlling good and bad Make-ups regardless, fitting In perfect slots is regarded higher purpose than Character A.S we hide prefer. Drawn on rarely seen 'Make Ups' flowing liquid Mercury, (No Groupings) run River Niles through A.S.s many Identities he Ink's. Few matching my Autistic necessity.

No real crossover Genre generic does A.S Group belong as either, 'either'. Yet Closer. Confusing maybe but, that was me breaking it down easily for you. Forgive me, I am Autistic Author.

Hovering in No Personality Groupings, other than his Autistic, his Character Shapes, No standstill Character he commits. He flows Open to what is heard; Around him. Debate is wrong, we enjoy (losing and winning) and don't debate further than our ((own, made up mind)).

This describes you Simon's Character, one guy living very different to his World. I believe this the Norm, I can Matilda myself no way other else.

Without given **Freewill** 1st place, higher peers try motivate stranger thinkers. An **unfair test** is just that **unfair.**

People who want you muster their Rules every step way, bad enough. I cannot help ask myself truthfully hand heart, friendship is made so sobbingly?

Answer: I want no part of fashionable friendship.

Birch staunched I only adopt hawkish stand off's.

A.S. joins your group through angst unease. Very clear to us '**our A.S. personalities,**' would only last **ayah long** with you, before start we heading home the Spectrum's Home. We up Sticks keeping you out, forever.

Either method adopted (both or singularly) would it is **clear, not keep** you **happy still.** A forever happiness A.S bound Always.

People look all the same in A.S.'s hills & Valleys and why different, is our Oxygen.

Fuzzy Bear 2.

'Fuzzy hearing' Is my notion moving forward creating a Fuzz, lure away deter those who don't think - gear, as me.

Fuzzy Hearing creates a confusion in us happy.

Fuzzy Hearing is just 2 words boiled down my very best describes; with what wherefore happens A.S.s Hearing.

Maintain Clean **Bells** & **Whistles** 'cleaned regularly', to A.S 's liking.

Much like people who build Kit Cars, draw plans up New Projects, making their newly designed Boats, Inventions, new Boardgames! Wants no part, **do with you,** (when his likening his ideas, till Shaped is his).

He can only reap a letting go once letting go **Standards** achieves.

In 14 Years.

In the **14 years** I have known, of my Diagnosis, ((**Mild Asperger's**)).

I have **Read only** really, '**2 Books** to date', along with Newspaper clippings columnists, reading about 'people just like me apparently', so I am coming from a place of Seeing, when **I am ready too see,** ready too learn, ((Similarity's)).. if at all. The One's I already know, 'of about' vacations in my found callings, perhaps.

Not taking on too much Understanding of others; before understanding Importantly 'who I am', with Mild Asperger's.

Therefore, not cheating my own Study Accurate, bit like believing in **God/Jesus** then seeing him in the Lights 'you thought you see him as' **as** the **youngster.** Not how now you really see 'him', boring this New knowledge.

Now you have adapted too a New founded '**Knowledge** in **Scriptures**', adopted In your found Studies discoveries awaiting discovering. Asperger's Syndrome Open and honest research, conclusions Summarises a good test, you took laid by you seeking accurate A.S answers you long.

I said I have **Read only 2 Books**, concerning a Condition on Spectrum, 'I have'.

So **Book 1:** mentioned. I recommend?

Titled: **Where there's** a **Bill there's** a **Way.** Author **Bill Furlong.** He's Autism. Bill is worthy of homage because his Authorship is worthy of your time.

Book 2: I recommend?

Titled: **The Curious Incident** of the **Dog** in the **Night-Time.** About a 15 year old boy whose names is Christopher. Has Asperger's Syndrome.

My mum introduced me to **book 2,** The Curious Incident.

This book, won a (Book of the Year). I liked this Novel for many good commonly found reasons. Nonetheless, from my perspective of A.S. If I may, Special I took home with me wasn't as much about the popularization found, I preferred presence what I read presented, what I found. Individuality catered.

Both these Books, 'shall do you lots of Good'. Care we Listen.

Autistic ((I told my Story)) in a different light; of hopefully others. That isn't sameness. We fight individuality we definition by.

Spectrum tell their, (own Personal Story), **Swimming Pools** same and different. My Cousin Autistic honest approaches, laying Mats, open Ears In earnest. One Chance too make Connection with a Spectrum Thinker, my hope suggestion, '**is you**', don't waste your time, trying too understand him fully.

Answers: laid down... his battle **shield**, tired lonely, bewildered. A.S Journey Syndrome tired, tied tired him down. Flow in this energy be Asperger once in a while. Leave more freedom learn Joyed. Hearing Acute furthering your journey an A.S, I come along Shaped.

Chapter 15.

Eye Contact.

Eye Contact (is hard making, as an **A.S**, especially), because we know, also **told.** It is Good too always keep 'Eye contact with People', whilst talking to Them. **On** one hand, **said.**

Said with **other hand...** we are also **told**, or **shunned,** for keeping this same Eye Contact', we were told ((was a good thing)).

By a **certain people**, who think you're **Staring** at **them.** (So you cannot Win). Is why a nervousness is inherit in A.S.'s, through mixed messages, he cannot Win.

Even if he tried 'another way', **someone who is** an **awkward customer towards you**, renders you weaker still. Looking away no Eye Contact confidence, comes next.

Suiting Up.

A **Suit** of **Armour** (I talk about), protects us Asperg, **same** suit of Armour a Normal person, (is in-used In).

We communicate ourselves over as this, (the **Normal** that **you are**).(In used In). Fore it is a communication you are familiar with.. 'However it is not the people we are'.

Yes we are Normal for your convenience, comfortable we are with this like holding our breath underwater. **Feeling** we must roll back to ourselves **soonish**, gasp... catch our breaths.

Pretending this is right way 'think, project', we feel uncomfortable at best. **Suited** in **Normal.** I am, Like a frogman/diver (all kitted up), with breathing apparatus, steers the murky waters. This is A.S in Normal suits - dished out.

Normal is not who we are. Where our blood runs true. It is just a Language we know, nothing more. Even when making strides an effort to conform too, what you'd (have us be). We cannot swim properly these waters, **just so** you are **kept happy**, the Normal amongst you.

Many people cannot understand, Asperger's our Natural.

Normal Asperger I shadow... I shadow what People 'want', crippling my true Work-ability disguised, for your benefit. Cause I Care. How you See me.

Bit like an Irishman speaking fast and you reading between the lines, it is **hard** at best. So you nod like you understood him. Cause you, Care.

Asperger's is my language (unto). Where we are from. Those who resign A.S. Growth. Meaning born Autistic, or developed into an Asperger's person as their person shaped told them. Shown all/part Signs. Asperger's Syndrome.

Like a Welshman can Speak normal English, **50%** can. **Welsh** is who these people are **1stly.** Though can speak (English Normal tongue), **again** for your **convenience...** though feel not as comfortable - his 1st, Welsh Native tongue, respected, they do free flow. Cause beloved Care.

So, consider Asperger's will and can **switch** from **A.S** with, being **considered Normal** often. Especially when finds himself in a situation he knows, his free flowing Asperger's, ((won't be welcome)). So he will again pretend for a convenience.

Though 'Normal Acting', **I do**!

Is popping a top button from my Shirt his wearing. 'Drawing on, turning into an **energy**', bestowed on me Autistic demanded. (He hasn't got). (I haven't got). Making us ill, drained, quick. Must find kick out hard, swims too Top his Asperger own... **Air.**

Our-minds understand a **language** 'we work fast for, work

fast In'.

It's common knowledge (accept another in our own), A.S Native Tongue.

So you may say, well if Asperger's can be Normal **like us**, what they hiding behind. Again, I tell you it is not the comfortable skin we live in.

We progress **once** accepted as **A.S.,** not you must conform too the regarded right, as you **say it**; must be **felt.**

Harsh on a **Mars** marsh-en crater, **is A.S.** suited in, **Normal.**

Chapter 16.

Finishing of my book, allowed to dry out naturally.

Job Centre don't like me Writing Books, One Adviser said to me: Simon you can't write books forever you know, yet it is where my Mind lives. I've struggled pushing more Time Out my friendly Team/Job Centre. And Grateful nonetheless.

I mention - I'd, Worked Hard on my, Second Books deliverance. And had come too far in deeper Waters too About Turn my Sacrifice. Way I see It, is I am Volunteering. If Not as an Author, on a Farm clearing Gutters, Sweeping Floors, no One knows.

It is all Volunteering Systematic too me.

I feel so Burnt Out Writing a Book without proper Backing. It's more of an Assignment these Days. I find the shame. I treat and say: (Yes), too everything in Life.

My next Job Centre Interview is on 18th March 2016. Today it is middle January 2016. By, Time you Read my book? Oh. Summer 2016 onward.

Still Reality is Reality. I am swimming in middle January here 2016, Today.

Frightened, I'll not finish in Time my (2nd Book) when 18th March 2016 rears an Ugly head. Finding Work other than an Author, is personally depressing. Torn Writing, before handing in my Rag, my Adviser Sally likes my many Ideas of (Creative Writing Courses at The Adult Learning Centre) in Guildford. Just one such Courses. Other Courses without rambling here! Oh. Word Processing many chose specifics. Though to date, I am fully booked with my English and Maths GCSE Course commitments at:

Guildford College. Coming up in September 2016.

So it is not all gloomy.

In-fact I have received much help from (Guildford Job Centre) as spoke too this point. Especially mainly Sally my P.A. she has taken dark clouds slowing my realistic mind; clean washing White Clouds rung, sliding pop whistles... here you go Simon. Very Grateful I got Sally. I am left much more options these days. Touchwood nothing changes.

I remain Captain Simon always wishing do well, though I usually find it is Others letting me down - when I am doing; what is called On me as (Wanted).

And this isn't helping my Condition A.S. I am sorry too say.

Usually this falls in line with such examples; Career prospects you put yourself on the Line for, with few Letters and Telephone calls, Exam results In waiting, answering my busied mind to Succeed. I am always prompt for Meetings, Appointments, chasing up Exam Results, chasing Enquiries, you wish were Returning deadlines I panicked, my commitment to be not Benefit, committed.

How I help out in my World is tailored accurately to my knowledge. Now my futures calling me further learning I am under going. **Same** as you'd under **go** an **Operation,** and everyone everybody is by your-side. It is this strength asking for. This strength I am in giving as Boy half Man.

Taking a Break when I meet you will you; love me whatever my state. Should I attach my pretend friend Image, pretend ego, charged at a Normal rates.

Let's try find Slack. You know Dogfish Boat fishing enjoying our best Memories. You and Me.

Let us part now dismissed Army's Platoon. My 'oath of allegiance' I thought we all took. **I promise** to do **my best God Country** & **Queen.** Immediate **Family** and **Friends** and **Readers.**

Cocoon Eggs.

My World as an A.S., Is always felt as uneasy among Others. Functioning only when we determine Conditions - ask, laid out. Not given this function, told we are Normal just like the rest.

Right wing Nature may say, we as A.S. shouldn't 'be any different', yet we are different. There is not an answer a man of closed Ears, will hear. He just sees it as (his physically alive isn't he), so he must be Normal. He must be Work capable, he must rally too our colours. Uncomfortable I function a Willingness Awkward forward with You, no passion performs with mindsets Company. My credence closing a Flower.

Humbled A.S. does of course (rally), (he's called Normal) expected of! he, tries and fails, your Normal Required, must be Like. Senses in him A.S., quietly cries.

Expected your happy he fits he, runs you your Normal by you, (he shuts down). Awkwardness presents every paw/ hair on an A.S. that made him originally glow A.S. naturalness now is enacting re-enactment, 'followings of Normal', that isn't Normal A.S not by a long margin.

Not understanding politics himself then, he is easily walked over. Politicians fore him or against lose/ win may forget his fight. Stronger nets try closing him down. They have power, not necessarily strength closing forward.

I am non changer what I once thought, many years/moons ago. Same person in thought today. Powers striking rich burdening message, of: **Change they want** - good or bad, Successful or broken-success, must ask! Is that what an A.S wants. Is that what Simon wants?

Writing this Book started as a scrambled framework, a bare Christmas Tree, I edited my adding/lessening extra decorations. Over long spans-ions nuggets joined together till - my happiness said. I can decorate no more.

Using my favourite saying 'less is more'. I feathered my

Oils In when editing, kept most my working word crafts short and sharp.

When a person writes this much with stacks in armoury remains, doesn't this say, there is - long way to-go before Asperger's is addressed correct.

Have you ever seen film named Cocoon, where they must be fragile with Alien Eggs, found in deeps of Ocean Waters, Dark blue.

Requiring Top security, hiding kept Cared for Eggs, Warm.

A.S. are those Eggs. Not wanting you tamper with what he sees as Normal. Vibe bubble he'll In use. Maintains his 1st asked for, language. Being as Normal as he can, pleases the other Normals. Dictates of stand by me definitions.

A, Likeness shadows on wall how every standard Normal, should mark himself down, critic - turns conditions Normal, turns conditions A.S.

Survival on Earth, this is how A.S. People 'Our **kind**', require the right cares entrusted, set lighting. Environment we work. Knowing what a Normal person is, what qualifies you categorize yourself as such. Something yes we are aware.

Our Normal senses Asperg Normal for sure is, Normal different from, Role modelled Normal.

A.S. I teach is my, Normal self. Educates 2 Normals existing, I division by/perhaps you division by.

Judged Autistic myself I can replica your Normal Identical.

Brother Normal looking back at me in my Mirror. Is only part my Story.

My quiet Autistic self goes unnoticed.

Scrambling walls of my Identity, I climb till I say 'that guy' stop - that guy is me.

Acting Normal I can do. Staying Normal I cannot. Writings of my Normal side enacted on me I can do, accepted as Normal springs land-sliding. Normal I lasted, too - first please You, (fell).

So losing friends again I am.

Short liked, Normal - I was, (falls). As quick as I came Normal acted.

I am losing Jobs again treated Normal. I acted out well. My real self carries less lies. Normal my head is heavy clots. My true Nature I am Autistic. I am now Rude towards another expected of seen Normal I am told I am, expected too walk as.

My Condition thunders only Autistic love. I whisper no connection Normal, my fight Grosses Struggle. Our time stays wasted burnt up changing Us to do your Better, is Our Worse Help.

Let us come together nurture all A.S. Compatriot's, from this point forward. Even all them without A.S.

A Planet, we can breathe fresh clean Air. ((Godliness; everywhere)).

Before we try mend Normals Help going any further.

Realize, our Nature calls. Natural demands Spectra dictates, I unfold.

Chapter 17.

Don't put your illiterates down, just don't.

People who make fun of illiterate people, dyslectic people, those who don't throw down Intelligence into Grammar & Spelling gauntlets many prefer to See. Mental compositions you shudder too accept, will often be pulled up harshly. Yet illiterates, concentrate same equal Intelligence often extra brighter other Activities they shine Good potential. Them regarded as intelligent, knock our Illiterates.

Displayed to 180 degree opposite side arch's, to not all be good at the same regressing ideals, yet showing more creative intelligence as one feature, where upon grammar is not their own strong point, double sides strong.

Myself, looking for what people can do with passion, not bullying senses of failure, over their Aura.

Them who took no time in School studying the English language (1) because they'd involved energies somewhere else at this time. (2) cause they didn't understand importance of perfect Grammar in a Society.

Others, Quick rejecting, misplacement of words, punctuation, spelling... Is always wrong - (mark the Writing) the message of what is said instead; trying adjusts, suggestive Teaching reaches him Merits.

I must admit becoming more proficient myself in good English, I have become - only through Interest of Books - I Write. And it is, dare I say painful, seeing mistakes these days, be it spelling, punctuation marks not selected in rhythm, or a daft daft mistake we all make when typing fast - or lazy today of mind.

I have Read, Articles - Letters - Emails, people who turnover as illiterate, and non so. With non judgemental eyes... I have found many times, more intelligence roaming in illiterates. A frustrated message they wish lay to perfect understanding English, so you shall, how you say, (get them).

Compared Scholars of English whose got all the tools reads beautifully, yet his weakness is his non passion dried up. I call this 'passion illiterate'. Just so you get top grades, not top personalized Spirited real Characters. Designs, free minded people show Arts, not grades so much they'd expect, or want.

The human eye pretty well knows what is good or trashy. Certificates are always a plus, yes. They're not forever the bee all end all. Qualified certificates coming out your ears, or just simple man of distilled passion yearned. I find you can never quite tell, one from other, beauty to be found in its many Scales, Intelligence divided.

Set beauty as feelings comfortable so, make the mistakes.

Is a better way learning, progressive, so start here.

Slow Limbo states of (mind, protect) growing we are.

Strict minds are necessary. Yet strict Teaching is not.

Avoided, wishing lower classed the same successes in life, (gave with), undertones to you.

Pronounced top people in Society, half cooked fish in their beefing up of own successes in your Success. Is almost like saying: I wish you well my fellow friend, and mind the huge step on your way out. Not to trip.

Told why the illiterate person, is comfortable to not shine as brightly as you, you must first work on befriending your students that falls not with strictness, yet teaches strict paths conducted, told not aggressively.

With this same concordance navigating Lessons you run.

Remember illiterates 'remained in a Slow Limbo', just for you so you may progress look fancy Oxford status. Them who knock Illiterates Nature as one subject covered, had not strengthened you, by not shining the other Clever You Are coming.

A 'strong reason' encouraging a love grammar English clean toffee nose before hands, is too (not, emphasis the strong placement on them) yet, work towards, help a dyslexia Intelligent. 'Otherwise you'll understand why they'll not develop'.

Mostly though it's not that illiterate people don't want to be the same Toffee you are, it's more in focus with loving gave equal no matter, your English Standards.

Chewing toffee you chew, we both look - damn fine.

Share your greatness this You & Me thing, my illiterate self, if I am - performing my way gone Solo. Intelligence then in a 50/50 split, carries wood.

Bring over an illiterate person walk bridges either side. Not feeling pressured lives, not on one side of bridge. Naturally brushing up his English, his Grammar bridge, sides... because 'he himself' prefers good Grammar.

Whilst kept freedom makes mistakes - ((if he so wishes)) under no pressure conditions better placed.

Signal cards making aware of Grammar moods (in him), today.

Less Ordinary to you is, our Extra Ordinaries to us.

Strict regimes followed as key first, when Caring key first, then teaching is this light, at end tunnel.

Therefore, it makes sense - relaxing In not always giving you your good clean (Student of English) language.

Had you not recognized illiterates moving back & forth

over either side of foots bridge, relaxed escapology, humans Spirit, relaxed approaches. Illiterates to be given River-Side Care.

So please help don't hinder wrongness you detest.

Most Illiterate people dyslectic people, call this as you shall, knew they were Crisp of Grammar/Spelling candidates somewhere in fighting out a brown paper bag. Just give them breathing space and, development will follow.

Stop trapping the wings of illiterates/dyslectics.

Illiterates place less emphasis, on having to get things so damn mighty right. They want to run you good English, with their correct reasons why they should. Proofing it's OK to Scribble and Oxford Cambridge yourself when! Care loved all their Bridges they came.

Relaxed, happy to learn of mistakes, adjusting still not afraid to make mistakes. Moving on grows (eventual), Great English.

And like those who take longer to pass their Driving Test, illiterates also are better (Drivers of English) grasped; better than most, better than All.

What's best obtained? (eventual knowledge) Is! without obscuring his mind with clutter, love his Scrabble side of crisp closeness expected of him.

Asked he reach striven heights 'when he's ready.'

Loving him healing. Loving him now. Loving him later.

He throws his illiterate name to one side, not so ashamed though, hang this title back around his neck.

Freedoms he infuses brought up Levels, bridge he walks. Freely on both sides. The Guidance Instructor volunteering help he'll give now.

Jumble Sale.

A book read (5), (10) years ago by you, made good reading, making best seller material, is little more than a book in a jumble sell these days.

The messages this certain book made spread, (was no longer). Your new direction of thought others hadn't heard of before.

Watching your book sell for 5p - the old lady with crippled hands, gave your book over to another. From distances of licking your own ice cream cone, you smiled to yourself - walking back home, knowing within the next hour, the old boy who you see buy your book, will be in your world soon.

Oh me? Well I'm jumping splashing my feet down the Seafront shoreline, holidaying my mind, taking a break. Moreover I'm rejoicing the freedoms - I had to just let go, deep sighing my personal relief.

Especially after sought book's, low popularity and high peaks, language tongue your readers captured, became apart of them. A thrown extra pillow behind the headboard.

Captured Reader read your book they became my heart. Strong strength is my Readers Happy for Me.

I am just an ordinary Man/boy wanting to Read any Reader's Books.

Write, placing no Anger easy stay with You, Intentions.

Something else here when writing books advice I lay in your lap, if I may, my Top Tip of day, novice swing intermediate myself, is this:

Bottled up messages, make you a good angry seated.

Not all things comfortably sat with you. Don't disregard bled Angry you, turn spin Anger - Good merciful Anger Good, a pancake well mixed.

Just don't dislike Anger, Others dislike You for harmless Anger. Try Embrace

your Anger, open Coke caps Beautiful let her Out. Anger doesn't have make you One Bad person, it can strengthen Help you. Gift Anger approachable Open Beautiful

Yourself. Tones of Open Good Anger don't just Dwell, don't frighten others, just say hey, this is Me. Display Anger look more favourable, advocate say your concern, tongue Good.

It is important, don't give all your best Ideas away before your book is Written, otherwise no true representation. Seeing reactions await with your (book), if a certain information is leaked by your own wagging tongue.

Discussing your book, you (Want) while (you Write) is not something, being honest with you here - I do; as an Author. 'And why I don't wag my Tongue'.

Take approaches you wish, I am just pointing out my warning signs, you subconsciously knew about - but needed me to resound out.

Good Ideas that are your property, will only remain Copyrighted - protected if you like - by keeping a 'strict tightening lid on, excitement whaling up inside you', is sat on.

Splitting you apart, you want Share, you got to tell somebody right, 'wrong, no **keep firm lids on it**'.

Or Ideas in your book, won't have kick same punch.

Bits & bobs.

A select handful say we will Reward those who Work Hard. Most do with no Reward, and manage a Smile. Good Men non stealing of good Ideas.

As an Author, I steer away publishing my Books via a Kindle device. Electronic book reader or any tech ebooks to begin, just because found is cheaper on your own pocket.

The payback, Oh soft kitten stuff to seeing your Real Book now in tow.

Ebooks great for later on publishing's, a month gone by.

Comparison, Oh none - seeing a Book, smelling and tickling the Spine of, you slaved tears Writer's pains you can then only start publishing in Ebook fashion, encourage you, keeps long chain on your wallet.

Your Book will not have feel good factor battle Scars, Good books require, If found quickly uploaded off your hard drive, to some Free publication taken your Work On, which didn't really take you all that long to Register.

Point I make is don't Sell Out Soul quickly, just to be Noticed gains of unwanted high ranking Friends.

Created in the changing World 'a book' where you started - you finished, Influence World around you 'undeterred you', whilst you took your time. Shaping a Name for yourself.

The best course of Action.

You lived through life 'unhurried', see goal line book finished not as important. While hurrying World gives You little time Open Man's Flower.

The man in the Village.

I dropped by my local Village Store Post-office earlier this morning, I've only lived here 8 months, time of typing. Surrey Hills... England.

Today's particular time I arrived, done all my usual things with the Post-office, like ask -can I pay my TV Licence here, instead paying Online, security stronger.

Annie is our Post Office lady, American, very Helpful.

I bought Milk at my Post-office store (3) 1 litre sizes.

I proceeded pay for my purchase along with 2 sandwiches bought to eat on my way home.

It wasn't the usual nice lady in our village Post-office today, this guy I'd not seen before - serving at the counter. He was of elderly discern, a werewolf type with long sideburns, if your forgive me, ready to pounce on any mistake I ran his way.

I paid via my Visa Electron card. After payment was authorized he removed my card, with no manners born in a

Village gentlemen you'd might expect.

He threw my Visa card down with the hardness in his voice, his fingertips exposed, like that of an Old born and bred Farmer, or stout Ale drinker. Wishing you felt his misery was unclear, A.S. I was feeling no Joy.

An Age 'he grew through' stuck in his Ways I felt no belonging whilst I gently closed Corner Stores post-office door behind me in Thank-yous, the bell on door ringing its traditional sound.

The Grumpy Man behind Counter takes -his Fill. Good Man, Idol - among other Villages mastering his Customers respect expected gave. Is correct, Traditional. It's right.

Befriending book guidelines? I show I am to Friendly, must work On my Manly Talk with Him, show him I am (One of Them) let me in your Club.

Slapping down my Electron card not worthy running his boat-lines - enshrined to his bootstraps - laces. I decree to Work Harder his Friendship.

Counter thumping my payment Card down without care he handed me my Goods: that's yours, that's yours, that's yours and that's yours. You could sense we hadn't bonded yet.

This probably Nice Store Man, Once you cracked the Code with him, only uses Grumpy disguises. He doesn't Owe No-Man Immediate divergence, his 'Rights' expresses him Grumpiness disposed when and where he pleases. A Man of Knowledge Opens his Road like this. This part grumpy Good Store-man took a disliking to Me. I stayed Happy.

He gave dare I say, Mr Bumble Character Oliver twist era. I respect people where I can with A.S. I understand life is like this.

Having Asperger's myself, your understand of my discomfiture, (to all people), running characters - I parallel no other way, still trying to Fit In. Rarely do I keep all folk Smiling. I last so long then stumble Autistic make shifting.

A.S. Speak on 'one' monotone level, strangers he not knows.

A.S. Speak on One Monotone Level.

Any disturbance to high & low frequencies, above below, from Kind speaking tones he surrounds himself in cotton wool. His first survival to sliding 'Angry spoke tones', Is from the least unsettling for Asperger divergence. Even smiling to keep you happy 'he's not OK.'

Adapted to a World where my frequencies don't Oscillate - 'must remain' is where Growth progress starts my slow Train moving, fishing around good, hard, fundamental foundations I Build. Useful Help Turned Out, Non Oscillated concentrations. My Offerings show my best Conduct left Alone.

The Oscillating World is too busy, with too many frequencies, all asking you Oscillate fit In with them, yet don't come from One Frequency Universal. They come from many separate Oscillations. I can't keep Changing my Frequency to suit every New person I meet, and so all too often Autistic man is maintaining his own Gifted Eggs, broken forever.

The Spectrum in question not Oscillating at All, sinks famous common Meltdowns, you heard of by now.

Any Oscillations taking place, given anytime Asperg Man, says! Is not a problem, just so as a long as - you know - he is the Oscillator only when left Alone, who tunes his (own senses).

I am lucky I have Mild Asperger's, you heard me say on Occasions, that my Meltdowns are controlled, easily over come, by such activities 'Writing Books', dispersing, pent melted anger as Achievement.

Be an Author not a Critique on others.

Council housing.

Council Housing, topic.

Council Housing should cater for Spectrum disorders

such as I, the same way as Community Sheltered housing, alike, will cater for a given Block of Flats, Street Areas bound by safe-nets.

As an example: the over 40's, over 55's, over 60's, receive! threshold levelled noise obeys, obtained.

'We told you - we need', and sure funny enough we do, require.

Lasting, 'undisturbed Buildings of happiness', is too follow through, already set out happinesses. Maintained this far.

Reaching to future maintained happinesses then must go further, A.S. and Autism housing requirement.

A.S. Autism flats and houses, Street areas, Towns, Cities and Rural fantastic buildings, Cottages - now to be built. Road Names allocated like:

Asperger Close. Autism Corner.

Spectrum Lane. Simon's Battle Road.

Bill's Way Meadow. Christopher Curious Close.

Hans Discoveries Way.

Yet more than this, isolated from Normal Society where our Normal way, gets more (elbow room).

'Required leniency of Noise in-particular', especially if pacifically specific asked, by I. Or him suffering.

Stopped doing Well moving on further I am, when others know these are my A.S rules locked In. Ignoring my gestures set-out, is like not re-cycling your rubbish correct - ignoring Spectrum's disorder, Want-ages.

Complaining as an A.S. Is my last last option. Often pushed limits I consider Unreasonable behaviour I proceed ask, they might adjust Please. With my pleasant tones spoke. Some neighbours don't know they're unreasonably Noisy. So ones got too approach, a certain Carefully.

Next follows a Grace period remaining Quiet only 2 Days, or was I nice enough? it Stopped altogether.

After this Grace period (hasn't held).

I Next send and sent my Neighbours many Complaint Letters, it gotten that Bad. Still Worded Carefully, biting thoughts I am tuning in turning out a Letter.

Awareness, I made of my Condition - Neighbours select handful - was likely you told the worst ones you thought were friends; were Neighbours misusing playing On the Normal! - they now know, (you're Not).

So telling someone I am A.S., only hampers with unreasonable types.

'These people shall do more' in aggravating your Asperg ways, now you silly told not thinking.

(The ones with a careless so what), forward of brothers on the Spectrum. Cares less for you than the thumping around down stairs his, aspired too. My silenced angry poles.

He Sees it as! it is his House, Flat, Apartment, he'll make as much Noise as he damn well Likes. Which is true I respect it is his Accommodation. While his World enters, heard in my Flat Above, an echo penetrating my 360 degrees therefore, not an Oscillation I am from.

He maintains forever, well 'it's my Flat' attitude - Quiet Arena my concentrated mind, eventually I excepts his large ego, nevertheless, I am losing development of my first Intentions! of how I wish too do well. Held discipline of what others say I should hark.

No respect is gave back to Man's Neighbour.

Calmly I complain, rarely. Although to-date - I moved home 7 times. Yes get that - 7 times in 5yrs.

I have handwritten (4 lots)- '3 page Letters', asking each neighbour brought into focus, said nicely. Please please in heaven's sake... stop thumping stop slamming doors, cupboards. It's not Normal behaviour. An 8.5 on my Richter scale.

Hence forth: I need unfold in an A.S. Building, people who are like me. Who understand me. My uncomfortable awkwardness, my unintended rudeness that can spill over, from time to time.

This is the **Community** of **people you Want,** as **A.S. Orientation** breeds **in you.**

You want Loud teenage youth?, then there should be Council Housing set aside (their kind), giving louder young, due respect also. The persons they choose - their followings.

Stages of life, you take Tailoring.

Separated by! - what Person's Write down, on 'his Housing forms'.

He/she, be given a choice, good starts your help.

In new changes Implemented - drafted & Signed.

You want Asperger Nightclub's you got it. Only Asperg's allowed In. Mixing mingling clinging to those who (understand you).

You want Clubrooms for Spectrum's - 'you got it', come on let us get political on this one.

Sign petitions over. Charity events do what it takes bring you & me up levels; we told each other we were.

You want Guitar Learning Halls for Asperg/Autism, (willing in Education).

Brill. So do I.

Let us really, (roll it out).

My A.S. life force.

My A.S Life Force: is weak; sensitive fragile; with strong. We break easy and why it is best surround yourself with ((your own kind)).

Ending book soon resting my battle shield.

Chapter 18.

Jobs I am considering at: Work-focused-Interviews. Attends every 3 months my E.S.A. entitlement.

I am in the ((W.r.a.g)) 'Work related activity group' although (Work Full-employment), is their end goal for me. I never fully understand why I must be pulled apart, mental ills, endure tests I must explain; already explained.

Agreements, arranged plans, re-setting re-setting forecasts, I mapped out in portfolios with our Job-centre-plus team.

Long grey letters, messy bedroom stockpiled with D.W.P Letters. Many varying letters, many varying Penned names, powers of (do words), easily rolled out as long as they're human rights, can't take tumbles, tumbled powers rolled out on (**less-able**).

Illness stamps, via authority roots over weak man's selfless assessed mind vulnerable condition. He has a better plan branded awkward, non magnetized to their ways branded now capable.

Branded for swings pushed in their favour fully charged on something, discounts a Place I function. I return Home collapse of my mind machine, powers me nothing they feel, yet I want to be Helpful.

I will say there is a running 'good side' to Job-centre-plus always however, a 50 /50 stigma regrettably. You going in with your ideas, plan forward then worrying making many ill, the 50 side alternative plan they keep true running colours - discounts your plans first forecast. Wet plate, dried straight away. Porcelain expected to always ring.

Working, Benefit recipients - Worked machine, (his ways) is when! he's asked for Special assistance, catering to his problems, and you see his from the genuine source makes (loved work), cared - pay. Not tactics same hard-work pays messages done, as other spectrum of 50. Full-Time-Work in my view shouldn't be the only End Goal. Voluntary Workers helping Taxpayers via Good, meaningful, construction, productive ways, plenty of good usage, is a way I conduct fairer and why Autistic I am prone to be up beat man plays fairer with human assistance.

(Campanology) Bell ringing in my Village I took Up where I live, told this kind of Work does not Qualify as Voluntary. And is said thought as an Outlet, more so. So something I enjoyed with provided Service to my community. Isn't making use of what I enjoy. And found this strange myself.

Personal Advisers at least the ones I was appointed always found - (very nice people).

I can't however say the same for **Security teams.** All in Blacks/white-shirts, chains keys bulging colours of chrome. Well turned-out men in Dr Martins at your local Job Centre - especially losing your way inside New Job Centres, asking politely 'I am Here for', or 'I got appointment with such/such.'

A Grunting noise to say his minimalist. A shrug of his shoulders curling his bottom lip, quietly saying do I look like I work here pal, as his name badge reflects - Security guard.

A Let down to his well turned out self. Most the time I try avoid asking them for help these days, cause it's like their doing you a dissatisfaction, the job they get a living wage for how might they pay tax, if there wasn't a job-centre-plus? Are we all in this together?

Bus Drivers are No better. I found they're Nice to you one minute, then turn on you dispelling all good Nice they were previous. Asking simple Tasks like I am about to dismount my Bus, I turn to the Driver, I call him by his First Name, make him feel at Home with me.

I notice he don't always like me calling him in less formal matters, so I revert back to Oh Thank-you Mr Bus Driver, then he thinks I'm treating him like a Nobody. Anything in between is half hearted. I am Autistic. I seek clarity in cut and dry, Yes and No.

I dismount my Bus. I say please what are the 2 Times after 15:30pm I can meet back at the (Bus Stop) and Catch my Return Journey Home. They speak something under their Voice at first like we're not meant ask such questions, and make you feel uneasy.

When I ask him (repeat) again please, his Tone is less than was before. Cutting through with him in a controlled manner, I say OK so that's the 16:05pm and the 17:15pm. He confirms with an almost don't Ask again ever, so always I am reluctant these days when confirming my Time Zones, how much Time I can spend (in One Place), so I know when my Bus is (due) In.

Where I live all Bus timetables are (Arrival Times) upon venturing out my front door.

Once In Guildford, my adopted Home town I like, all Bus journeys taking me back home are (Departure Times), so constantly you must convert each way (all times) wherever you Are.

So Arrival times/Departure times. Takes some getting use to. Buses are unpredictable living in a Village. Even when some claim to the Contrary.

Any Job I get, Full Time Work, Voluntary Work, or making my Way back and fourth in College Courses I enrol, creates no stable guarantee for any Employer, and why I felt wasting money on Bus fares waiting 20 minutes to up to 2hrs for a Bus you try predict will (turn up on Time), doesn't (not always). Then once Bus Arrives I am Guaranteed at least 1hr 20 minutes Bus journeying. Time I reach my destination I am drained already before beginning a mandatory Job of another's choosing. This is why I'd Happily Volunteer in my Local Village Church working up to 16hours/40 hours per one week or making up Hours in Self employment Interests I can Hobby your way, make Coffee Tables for Instance - Sell them On. Paint people's Gates, Walk their Dogs, cut down Trees, become Village Carpenter handyman, help Elderly jobs I can do free. You get the Idea.

This way Work I do, 'is Flexible'. Work with my condition Asperger's Syndrome. Tailoring my own hours I give back to my Society this means it is not unfair on an Employer those times I can't Work. Or am lessened man hours my, many problems I do encounter.

I'll happily waste my time and yours, giving you my documented accounts, painful mental ills dedicating my whole life explaining - not accepted, as Simon A.S.

My end goals may be (Voluntary), (self employment), (full time work) built with my terms helped along (not) Changing me. Working in a freelance way possibly, and why Writing books is my direction I am tapped into.

I am seriously contemplating taking 3 A Levels at College, requiring A-B-B Grades so I may further my Study of Music, or simply Subjects of Interest to

me - as an Undergraduate, at the University of Surrey, or College of Music.

Firstly I must meet Entry Level Certification. So I am currently in the process of waiting on (results) an assessment I took at Guildford College the other day, so they know themselves the Level of my Maths & English core Subjects, placement in Pre-GCSE or without the Pre. They decide best for me. 2 Subjects road mapping me loose laid structures so I may relax awhile. Before deciding the each next step, forward Action plan.

Qualifying myself at University or College doesn't matter so much which, Opens doorways to (Full Time Employment), paid for something I enjoy very much.

For small while voluntary worked at my local Church in Village Bell-ringing, couple hours on a Friday, then I retreat home, spending my last energies as Author Simon. Always in fear my benefits will end, meaning no way to publish.

Plans were, and currently are being (drawn up), that

works with my Asperger's in a fairer way to previous Job-centre encounters. That's not to say (Job centre - remains) understanding fair - you're always not given - your own plateau.

My old (Personal Adviser Lisa) at Havant Job-centre-plus in Hampshire turned around me saying Simon, would you consider say Self-employment? I explained I was Yes, happy breaching considerations moving this way and were Interested please.

I explained my 1st Book, (Plain Truth), wasn't brilliant, in fact it was a hard read for most Normal people. Critiquing myself harshly cause I get mixed up jumbled up words, so the Grammar king in me is some what flawed, and maybe if I can find the strength I'd like to re edit my first book one day, making it more reader friendly.

I do make my apologies book 1 Plain Truth, leaving you the reader awkward uncomfortable (for me). I did so with an intention showing language barriers.

We tend to as A.S ((disappoint and please)) the masses. Compensating relieve in us, burdens one as greater.

And so it stands Justified - takes a bed of mistakes - before the Asperger man shows his high functioning self. Stunned amendments amazing you not too so much shock.

Praying I served you justice I walked my tightrope in book 2 - today with you.

My first book is on Amazon.co.uk However, due to my first book seemingly carrying a flop message with persons, I (gave) my book priced at £7.95p at the time.

So if it was said my 'first book', serves as a reminder the heavy cumbersome message I am. Just think how hard Autism people live this trodden down feeling, ((they're no good)), they're no confidence. Then in futures time prevailing, your understand all living under a Spectrum disorder - can display Failures, Successes, wherever they choose - not knowing who'll get the divided sides of you - this day - yesterday - tomorrow.

There are 2 Groups on E.S.A. - the benefit I am in receipt of - (WRAG, Work Related Activity Group) or (Support Group).

The group I am in, WRAG.

(Alternative Thinking) is a symptom of A.S. So look here, when asking why I'm so set, work from my own toolbox labelled Simon's tools - etched in all my tools, security reasons not to lose these looked after tools (I carry).

Jobs I am ready to consider, I don't want to lose my E.S.A Entitlement are: followed list below, in bit.

Ideally I'd not rather go down the route of Full Time Work Employment even though this is what our Government (chip away at you) - saying this is what we want for you. Cold wet fish feeling, smirking the glee.

Rather than coming with fairer outcomes - my Asperger's stands - a better way, too survival.

Misunderstood ways. Others I'm forced Work with (don't understand me). Even when said look after this guy he is an Aspie relieves me no appetite. Worked mandatory, is not given powers freelancing A.S. Showing promise, non mental illnesses required please.

I personally think Forcing said Person into a Job - to (take any Job is wrong). Just keeping Taxpayers' regarded one way rules, they're on lock-down under brokered in as freedoms, the spirit of man smiling is hemmed in - not to find new ways he'll expand.

Forever dogged - volunteering his help. He gave willingly in life and was mocked. Not working to pay tax - working only to (help), he then qualifies, ((tax paid in by effort)) surely.

Since money is distributed in mind warping mysterious tunnels, so does it not stand to ground him paying tax for others. Why grumble hold bitterness?

Is it not Earned - by any receiver who volunteered - work completed, he gave back (put In) to Society.

Taxpayer gave, sure. Yet Volunteer spends money granted to his honest simple ways, not dogged if Spencer or Jane got more than him. And when simple volunteer helped out, yes he spent other taxpayers' money, and when he did, he helped enterprise businesses he spent freely given handed back, handed over. Everything is temporary. It is just a method we pay by, encourage Openness.

Do Employers, who pay employees, not pay their tax (for them), given handed to government? Do I, as a volunteer not work with businesses, and take on work for them freely volunteering?

Are we (the simplest workers), punished simply cause we See the Jobs required of us, get on complete the job tasked and do a better job, with him who was jobbed as paying tax? Volunteers help Jobs done along quicker, so more Tax is left with Governments.

We are jobbed as using heart and spirit, care and attention to detail a paid man cannot always give.

Results compulsory Jobbed = heartless manufactured Products. Label stamped, cellophaned, boxed. Repeat.

With no more care than to 'make money'. Those making the big buck built Products/Goods - not made to last. (We're told that is OK).

Good paying citizens can't see the reality of the money spinning machines, the high bosses just paper-tape over (closer inspections), easily gift-wrapped as ruled within the boundaries of law. The driving force is (tax paid) taking directions, profound of high seats, - all else is scraps - seagulls given.

Great - they who are 'worked' (not to care), work to pull in money, a bad name attached, much later.

Shoddy Craftsmanship so to keep up on demands.

They lose hand over fist Capital invested back into the business (cause no ones) coming back to them. Wasted time and effort builds Products, manufacture Goods - not lasting. Materials scrapped early.

When our ((volunteering guy)) paying (no tax) receiving 'said handouts' had done a better job, did it freely not to - make gains - he remained poor, yet kept his skills tuned helping the masses.

Only to be told, he's a scrounger of his own thought through ways. Soul dedication he gave each and every Job satisfaction turn Merits.

Happy there are more ways to fry fish achieving more flavours on palette - is done via experimentally.

Found only when (not dogged), found only when (backed by - people's power) find a reached KFC secret recipe mama.

I cannot turn my own temperament Warmth's up - fearing everyone's regulated. Only those who work hard are rewarded, any form of work-hard methods I use other than, (this is the only way), is quickly snapped off line - like dead seaweed.

How can might that promote healthy business relationships catered for the freer of men? Oh it is not fair - you are saying. Life isn't fair, so lose your own principles!

Born rich privileged they maybe are born with Values laid on a plate for them. All they are required do, is wear the dictating sandals and pull on an already taught fishing line. The strengths job made from, silk Slippers.

Simpler man unaware of his human rights. They worse for ware are reeled away, inch by slow unnoticeable inch. He doesn't notice he is being (Changed). His now mouldings cast not of man's Sunnier days looking back once remembered.

Whilst those making efforts paying in their help to Society Voluntary manners, rendered, non taxpaying status.

All I can do is say (look) why don't you settle me as Voluntary, earn my Benefit's where I am put in a driving seat. Not called in for any-more romantic Job-focused-Interviews at Jobs-centre-plus. Say we came to an agreement, that this here will be your Job rest of your life Simon.

If (change in me) is a seeker, in you by you!, you're hypothetical to say, (change in you, doesn't want too change either). So correct Career roots I admired you for, a difference of man's mind methodology we divide our tumbles is always one stunted to dominate over another. Principles I obtained, you obtained, is not equality at Work. Fore I carried on admiring your Roots, whilst explaining I still See things different.

Kept same Voluntary Jobs until, better happier places of Work becomes found, happiness being 1st Port of call. Options Liberated. Full Time/Voluntary should be Man's own Option. Not his shamefulness.

You say to me: well going to work Voluntary Simon you may as well go in Work Full time! Again you're enemy (for Change). We don't want Change.

Oh (what we want, don't count). I see, we don't get choices. We get what is gave. So than Powers are greater than Principles. I find sadness this shame.

Healthy Individual is built on compassion and so is his Entrepreneurship humanity Rights. Man abides (the obeys) sure. Principles wrapped around a system of monetary, is 'your best answer' why we are ((forced ill)), for thinking in terms A.S. ways.

Gaining Employment = a lot of: more paperwork turning changing over mindsets, with no Ambition empathy driving my own directions forward no guarantee has any Employer taking me On, getting a guaranteed package. (Flexible Working) would be my best Option regarding a very good Action Plan, forward. Why declined am I enthusiasm, I guarantee Success?

Self suffocating Interests, such mind-bending (housing rent forms), paying rent direct out my wages, if in Full-time Job. This is no guarantees of my commitments, work not interesting me or how long it'll be before I'm - turfed out, on my ear as an... A.S dedicated theorist.

Commitments, Voluntary work I say I can do, or (Flexible Work) gives me that all Important Life Jacket I have more than followed as Seeker required. Gives you commitments I'm sustaining too. And no changing or filling out ((more forms)) if things go wrong.

Voluntary Work or (Flexible Work) is what I hammer home is my A.S requirements. As you know Full time Work is the End Goal seeking of many wanted for me. However, I find it strange that an agreement cannot be reached since I am prepared to Work a Voluntary work or Flexible Work from up to 16hours, build to 40 hours. And more working hours on top. Time sheets built on - my health, monitored this week.

There's no guarantee I'll get on with people I'm placed with - and teamwork is demanded of this factor (in life, played out Full Employment).

So (staying Voluntary) doing my bit in the World, is doing a Job, 'the same as Employment offers', (just paper money, sets us apart).

So look different. So look yes sure - I am A.S.

It is up-setting, there are many people diagnosed with A.S. who are (ashamed to be called A.S.s) yet here I am, unashamed of who I am, and told I almost run as Normal, and punished when I don't.

So look sure I'll take a risk of Full-time Employment.

It is a risk taking on me Full-time Employed. So your best chance and my best chance is established finding me Full-time Work where I am just left Alone. Completely on my own. (Flexible hours), built strong freelancing. Then we can strike a deal and move forward.

All Self-employment Ideas I have set in motion (to-date) is more wasted effort you're prepared to take away (my self educating ways). 1000's of pounds I invested Guitar Musicianship courses, Projects I made helping musicians 'via Guitar Aids' I crafted from Wood. Qualified City and Guilds Carpenter and Joiner, disjointed - because I come Voluntary my End goal.

Self-employment is risky especially for 1st time Comer like I, to this Game.

Do I 'Sign Back On' when every time I have a bad Week bad Month bad Year, not able pay Rent, Council Tax, and so On? Should I not be adventurous show Courage show Keen - based on politics where, my otherwise good Works I produce is your Gain. Shunned on pretty smiles at the Job-centre although they do care I believe, there is nothing making me feel connection.

Projects 'in the ready' set to my small business plan templates, all discussed with Job-centre-plus. Inclusive is working with (Enterprise First). ((All wasted)), cause no guarantee is my Autistic backbone granted 'Backing' would require built A.S. Flexible.

I make my concessions to You, willing put myself out for you. Not budging laid Issues not one inch, hard headiness, mixed with Care we both can be found A.S or N.T. Nothing is completely weighed strong.

Comes up with no concession working under One Umbrella.

I suggested Voluntary Work even though I'd rather be at Home Educating myself on Guitar/Writing Books. Or like making ((Guitar Aid Projects)), benefiting students of my Acoustics Guitar World. This work talked through all backslid-en through the years. You already know.

Qualifications are no longer Important with Me for I once was following correct Career Paths look where that got Me, people disliking 'me', Apprentice of the Year presented my Tankard at Awards Night. People weren't happy for my Achievements my Progress. It actually hinders when doing, too Well. Hard work I gave. 'Lost'. Then you say hard workers shall be rewarded. Tallied up Autistic not sure, I share logic you purport.

Asked by my Governance to do Well for Them, so fixed on the Prize. You see my Keenness kept Fighting tired, knowing my own principled mind tells me, cut the Winners some slack. I don't require make you proof of my Winning, you said my Job is of a Simple man. So I won just below the poverty line, to fit In. Reminded no one likes a smart Alex.

I shall gain Qualifications again for You and Me. Steer me where I want to be. Where you want Me be - it is said. Though pushed for Greatness asked for, this time I shall not - fore when gave You, I progress No further. Too many dangling Carrots, wastes my Time.

I have given up being. The best in my areas my arena.

Here is a Jobs list, considered Mental health not added. Truthfully I'd rather Work Alone.

I Sign with my Fountain Pen, held Help.

I will do any of the following Jobs Voluntary - Full-time employment - Flexible Employment.

So here is my list - follows next:

Simon's job list:

In no particular Order.

1. Leaflet Distributor:

For any Parties - don't mind I'll just do it.

Simon's party's below Rain or Sunshine help you on deliveries:

Labour - Lib democrat - Greens - U.k.i.p and so fourth.

Call me.

2. Book Author.

Write books Subjects Topics: Asperger's/Guitar.

Help those with no hope. Helps do a Job I take enjoyment.

Selling my books I make no profit made by me, Charity Raising Money, so seen as productive good works Coming your way.

3. Write books on Guitar:

Helping those with Special difficulties, Beginners, Intermediates, Advanced levels. Thus helping me, (not seeing, past work I invested) - over £9,000 going to waste educational Dvds and Books sitting in unused quietness my living-room on shelves. Only on show pretty cause no conclusion was met with agreement - I poured mass efforts into Once upon a time.

Is certain destroying walking past your Acoustic/ Electric Guitar every single day knowing you can't fully commit the way you'd like for fear of Job-centre moving you away - directions from, already once instilled in you. So what do you do? You write books - expressing one's emotion.

Thus sharing head knowledge, I wilfully help out fields of Guitarists. In turn they help my circle.

Even though at my age 43, my body fails me slower, my mind is quick.

What has not failed me is my own enthusiasm for all things musically played as Instruments. My axe of choice Acoustic Guitar.

The One asset that's alive kicks in me - remains my over active brain, healthy good knowledge I can lay with Guitarists. Rusty knowledge I've endured, cause my 1st keen directions - kept distracted, asking what I'm doing look for work.

Ready too Mig/Tig weld I am - mild steel, over all remaining rusted out past educations, once strong in me. Only to have too go back through - theory and practice sessions with no guarantees the gov will back you. An eternal circle of rust jobs, for ever patched makes your advancements slip back, rich-only in rust red dust oxide.

Way you must 'keep up, playing Guitar', spraying rust resistant paint, on all repairs of - kept up educations bore in you, drummed in you, once lost, now maintaining, with no further government distraction rusts, throwing you off.

Forgetting taught educations you took on board. Your harbours mind needs remain strong - so new educations, take root bind layered grips on old foundations in place. Velcro New on Old. With Old on New. Then mixing it up with Measure.

Finding yourself battling this craziness. Educations you

surrendered to all else on hold. Including your Social life, was your way of contributing to a world of many warps then told, No Wrong - cause study 16 hours a day isn't gov policy and you must get a job. Meaning your dedications with Arts of Musicianship are never studied, then practised with Vigor.

If not for me, help others in your future who are driven by the Arts. Time ticking, never giving them/me 'backing'. Ours yours, enthusiasm - destroyed.

A Musician. Writer. An Artist - freelanced advocated freedoms concentration, he must reach - ought be left with him/you. (should it not - this way - be?).

Aiming more pacifically specific, to an audience with those not realising they (have a gift). Many people through their lives have made them feel, they're unable to do Well - just plain worthless.

The way I try help out combats the (**I can't dos**), not because I have to, cause I want to.

4. Guitar Teacher.

Working with anyone not considered Normal gladly. (People high functioning yet with disorders) like me - are easier attuned Students to tap friendships, where upon they can take my teaching reigns - at times of excellence.

Most Times our disorderly friends cover up motor skills, (harnessing gifted truth). I'm afraid is harder - most their life kept down, they can't use such skills, shining with intelligence like Normals. Those with extra ambitious drives don't want you dampening their arenas - so someone's got take the credit - usually is them.

A certain credence I am, those prescribed like me - lets others trample 'over us', with whom caring sensitivity ranges stronghold of wavelengths found in us. Always denied a buffering look good, so those who don't care who they hurt, 'get higher,' for all books written marks only high status. All should share a Wealth a chance - do Well.

I am here to mend broken paths, working with Learning

difficulties - Mentally disadvantaged - Mentally handicapped. Simply disadvantaged full-stop. (Try me, I'm approachable).

5. Copy Editing & or **Proof Reading** Courses.

A way to earn my benefits, 'provides Job Resulting', I Volunteer happy, leads to Full-time Employment, do this Course: Job-centre send me on - Right.

Again I will pack my lunch each day, seeing a College Course through.

This sort of work will suit me down to ground, especially left alone, working from Home preferred. Courses designed packaged for home study.

A Job I am able to do, enjoy do.

6. Making useful Carpentry - Aids at **Home.**

For Guitarists of all ilk, Normal Guitarists in all, Private/Commercial/ Industrial uses/. Guitar Aids I can supply to Universities & Colleges all over the World, promising you benefit - all Music Professors, Lecturers & Students.

By my hand, Projects Ideas, I make Guitar life simpler, less time consuming. I give you more life energy back progressing you harder, further than you required. Spoils for choice. Such Projects are:

Guitar Coffee Tables: large scaled size (Fret boards) 'Guitar Necks' (blown up bigger) easier on Eyes. Running through horizontal centre beautifully crafted coffee table top - work surface.

This coffee table elevates 'up' from its standard flat position, up to the angles of 45 degrees where most things become readable.

Scales, Riffs & Licks, that boggle the very adapt now mapped out visually in front of you for your own easier usages.

Leaving you no awkward Clip Folders and folders of mind scrambling - Riffs - Licks - Melody's - Solos, balanced on (one knee). Now you simply arrange your own Song

Compositions, leaving (your pens) less work - less ink.

Guitarist grateful - I scaled out, workable (Scale Patterns) frightening, complex Guitarists work with.

Such as: ((Major and Minor)) - Diatonic - Pentatonic, Scales.

((Starter Scales)), I designed inventiveness 'in the Open positions', near the 'nut area'. Headstock areas on your guitar. These Starter Scales allow you to traverse through any given 'Major or Minor Keys' which adds extra thinking out the box. Not stuck to learning (new Keys or Scales) in only one default area of Guitar's Neck. Now you're free to roam, with more options at your disposal.

((Blue Scales)) many scales, mapping the sometimes complex arenas of your Guitar's neck.

A drop, from a waters ocean, before you're ready for complicated Scales you'll work with one day. Hybrid Scales - Melodic Scales, all the various ((**Modes**)) of the **Ionian:** The Mother of Parent Scales is born from basic, Chromatic 12 to 13 Note Scales.

I will Guide You, wherever you Struggle, for I am a Struggler no different.

I Introduce learning at your pace, without rattling on.

Here is one more example of ((Guitar Aids)) I draft up - design - then Craft helping the Musician out:

Such as: **Right Rhythm (**hand**). Hand-boards** is another Project I build depending on the leverage I'm given here, is more I will Help out In ways I bring.

There's a big Market out there to explore Projects, I can earn my benefits via, or you can pay me in, full time Job - not fussed.

Fought with painful outcomes 'to achieve results'. Great achievers strive, working with my humanity, giving too big of (what I can do), if growth starts as **less is more**, attitude I as one within Work.

Better laying big plans than non. Promise more than you

can deliver - whilst remaining striven. A.S.'s relieve the over flux this way.

Possibility's are yes, endless.

So let us move on, these are only ideas I'm toying with, floating with you.

And by no means Detailed, till born Interest is shaking hands with me.

((The Right **Rhythm hand. Hand boards**)) simply: Strumming Ideas, Sequences, Patterns, Chord progressions - designs of useful.

Building your 'Musical Guitar Chops', a place you can call Home tap into my designs, Right Rhythm hand - Hand boards, I bring you a purpose.

Play along with your C.D.s at Home Pick up your Acoustic Guitar - Key In with Music you love. Playing Accompaniment be apart of an Ensemble. Jam with your Guitar Buddy now my Right hand Rhythm Aids are Aiding you.

I shall always have many other Projects, I can sit with you when the times are right. Too much description for this book (so let's leave it there).

7. A Delivery Driver.

So another Job I can do walking away from all jobs I suggested so far becoming Driver.

I have a full car driving licence clean passed my 'PASS PLUS'. (Positive Driving Course) with an Approved Driving Instructor, D.S.A.

I Voluntarily or Employed go into certain **Delivery** driver **jobs**, earning benefit by being this full time driver - if left alone please.

Or as Harvey Keitel said brill Actor, in a film called **From Dusk** till **Dawn**, 'I'm a Truck Driver, look outside your door in parking lot, you see a large recreational vehicle (that's mine). In order I drive that legally, you need a (class 2 driver's licence).

This bar is for truck drivers - (you say). Well I am a truck-driver and these are my friends.'

Barmen announces: ('welcome to the titty twister) - at the Titty Twisters bar.'

So OK. What **kind** of delivery driver you want to be Simon?

Err-rm: Pizza delivery - Car parts delivery - Parcel force deliveries - Courier driver - Parcel delivery - Florist delivery - Super Market delivery - Carpet delivery - Removals delivery - e.t.c & so on.

8. A Job in **Religion**.

So Happy to consider helping out in Churches.

Become a **Monk** or **Friar**.

Spiritualism Church - help out Voluntary. Open to suggestions.

Church of England Anglican, Christian, Baptist, Catholic, Methodist, Evangelist Churches, so on, e.t.c

I'll work with most Church types depending on beliefs I hold - they allow/not allow, you see.

Not here change or rub shoulders (in Church) so I fit in.

I ask only acceptance.

Happy Promote Church events in leaflets handed out.

Anything centred around the: '**Word** of **God**.'

Spreading Lord's Happiness. Work he ask relieved - sovereign (Lord's) suffering. He didn't die for us/me, without glory given back. Amen.

Growth slowly with my Lord, I am patient I'm ready.

Update: currently Volunteering my service Church (**Bell-ringing**) in my Village Surrey England.

7.30pm - 9pm is practice nights. Our Church has 6 Bells in the Tower.

I met some great people here in Surrey. Joshua my friend teaches Campanology Ringing Bells at our local Church.

Guy is our Tower Master - lovely man.

New Update: Due to Campanology not considered as 'Volt Work', I had to give up Bell ringing. Pressed, look something elsewhere - they declare as (Volt).

Disheartened, Bell ringing helped me take (activity) in Village.

And gave me an Outlet.

9. Work with **Spectrum Disorders:**

A.S/Autism. Work in say old/young people's Home.

Homes for (all Spectrum disorders) young or old.

10. Join the **Services:**

Army. Navy. E.t.c. In rolls I am able undertake, if left alone.

11. Become an **M.P.** (Non official role).

Member in government as a representative of A.S./Autism/ Disorders, and so on. Study Politics at University.

12. Work Voluntary in **Charity Shop.**

13. Wash Cars Voluntary. Or in self Employment.

14. Fisherman.

Boat fisherman. Merchant fisherman. Charter boat fisherman.

Trawler boat fisherman.

Job where I'm at Sea, left alone not governed.

Allowed to freely (be myself), within reason. Keep my nose clean, respect my skipper.

Just don't want all too familiar patterns appears after rhetorical again. Others saying ((they can't work with me)) - for ways I think.

Team me up with a Skipper who is tough - caring too - gets the jobs done, like a granddad role model loyalty.

So there was a **List** of **Jobs** I said I can do, although my body's pains these days, smiling, saying freely OK - this what I help do.

I can't help my Awkwardness cramping me, follow (how you'd like I grow) always hinders me an awkward, walk in me.

Helping out as you, deem (I try) - just remember please 'this is your dream - your interests'. My voluntary, Flexible Work powers, remains not commitment I can run out tomorrow conveyancing allowance set Castles ((Life for myself)).

Chapter 19.

My Work-focused-Interview.

On 26th June 14 at 15:35 hours.

I said too Lisa my P. A., look Lisa (I think you know) my stand, honestly frankly I'd rather not Work, for it governs too much already, work patterns not of my accord. Nothing is ever given back where a Man can feel real Control, dampening on his larger Spirit. Hard Work requires you give Man's own Nature Back. You need to Enrich a Man's Strength, so Hard Work is Skittles he knocks down with Ease. Too many Clamp downs on Man's Soul sits illogical, within me. Where my Work pays, is friendship 1st.

With less mandatory friendship.

Come to some drawn up step by step agreement, that those governing us say hey look Simon you are happy with Voluntary Work right? A means to earn your benefit. You have ((declared)) many times (**Fle**xible Work - **Fle**xible Hours), is a route to leave benefits behind. Then look we'll not hold you up any further with 'Work Focused Interviews' every 3 months, at this Platform my friend. That generally we do know you're not **focused In**, the Time it wastes my **Action Plan** already on track. Let's not string out yours and my Time. We know this Game, so let's play a good game, a fair game. Stale-Mate isn't our Game Over, it is - best of 3 Remember.

Instead set up '**Vol**untary Focused Interviews', **Fle**xible Focused Interviews, as End goal Achievement. Give control back to Man. Voluntary Jobs he completes a range of ways on Rota. In Shifts. New powers, (People Advertising) outside their front Doors - Privately Commercial or Industrial, Voluntary Workers they bring out the Cold.

No set Hours you must take, (choices), all our Volunteer must Show is 40 hours of scheduled Work, he's found on his own Merit, off his own Back. So One Week he could be Mowing Lawns 9 hrs, cleaning Mrs Johnson's Attic out 3 hrs, thus helping Mrs Johnson get on with Jobs in her own Self Employed Business she runs, enabling discipline deadlines met, now Mrs Johnson isn't split apart with Personal chores I do for her, and Running a Business.

This all means She's, Mrs Johnson Is, earning pulling In more money. Now dedication to her own Business gets her full attention, which In turn is more Tax Collected from her contributing, and me Volunteering, her Healthy Business good Drive.

Volunteer waves bye bye to Mrs Johnson, and Thanks her for her Rose hip tea, and finds more Voluntary Work, so he can Report back, phone In at Job Centre HQ another Job Ticked. Mrs Johnson Emails Jobcentre-plus quickly, confirms Simon stopped by, and Jobcentre is Happy.

Volunteer continues a Free unburdened life, built on his free mind. He maintains good Relationships with his Customers and Jobcentreplus team, so they always know where he is, without feeling hounded.

Today I search out extra Voluntary Work so I make 40hrs an easy crossing line. I find Work today in my Village. Mrs Lacey, who is Elderly, I phone her before I arrive not to startle, I complete 2hrs Ironing - 6hrs I spend cleaning out her 5ft Aquarium Fish Tank she loves dearly. I also fix her (fish pump) which just required a New Starter Switch, easily bought at Fish World round Corner. While I am there I buy 2 Budgerigar Honey seed sticks, a new Iodine block and One New Mirror one of her Birds pecked off before. I ring Mrs Lacey's door bell in rhythm we agreed on, so she knows it's (me), she lets me back In. I tidy up Jobs I started, and watch a (film) with her bringing me to a 10hr Day. Mrs Lacey is elderly so Jobcentre agree to phone her, and check Simon completed chores as drafted.

I wave bye bye Mrs Lacey and feed her Cat before I leave her safe. I make her a nice Cup of Tea, and leave plenty of Water in Kettle, so she don't need keep Refilling.

Today I find Voluntary work in my Church welcoming New Arrivals to their Pews, Seats. I hand them out a Programme booklet so they may follow along Singing Hymns. I run a small speech 3 to 4 passages out my own Bible, then return Welcoming people In at my Churches Door. Everyone goes Home, at 13:30hrs, by this time I've clocked myself 4 hours Voluntary Work.

At 14:30hours I agree with my Vicar to stay On, and help out with extra Chores. Big Wedding Today booked - (I do so) the Wedding finishes, I brush up the confetti, refill Holy water font, I say a Prayer before thanking my fellow Church goers. We shake hands, I go Home and run a Nice 8hrs Today Voluntary Work.

I am 10 hours short still, with only 3 days left to meet Voluntary Work required of me, so after building a Log book Voluntary Customers I Serve, I find it easy to make my last 10hrs Up. So I call On my friends Mr and Mrs Oakley, who today have just the Job for (me). I clean out the Stables, refill the Troughs, and learn how to re-Shoe a horse and tie her saddles. I make 5hrs today and Mr Oakley phones Jobcentreplus reassuring I made adequate progress.

I gander through my Customers' Log book, I built over 14 months. Today I decide finish my last 5hrs Voluntary, Answering telephones at Jobcentreplus also Welcoming In benefit Claimants, showing them help, in Jobs they Search.

Volunteers (Working for Taxpayers), who themselves say we're not a Problem. Happy in Full employment, Self employment are those who have their Helpers us Volunteers. Throw some earnest fun In. Throw some Spice in, and People Communication is less people Angry, less people Screaming around in Angry Cars.

Full-Time employment, might be something considered if and when he/I Wishes, In the Mean Time if the Man specifically calls to you he'll stay Voluntary all his Life, then I say Jolly Good Show.

Fulfilment - Jobs en-worked, Volunteers Way, (he) Agrees.

College Courses his taken Interest he took wilfully,

therefore you're under no illusion to agreements you're signed up to. The way you contribute your own plan forward, your society's structured promise.

Our (Voluntary Interviews) needn't not drag me out, spend £8 each time on Travel expenses - just to reach our Job centres location. We may instead conduct an Interview (over the telephone), saving all Money.

Saving all dignity.

Travel Expenses only incur (I pay - I give), handed over to more Mr bus drivers.

In turn, creating more wealth, fascinating ways in which it keeps big businesses thriving, especially large Bus Company's making every penny count.

They then, ((bus drivers)), are taxed on their Weekly wages and somewhere in all the tax handed back collected - ((is my Bus Fare I paid)) each time. So boosting, profits margin for both Bus Company and Gov tax collections. Is a good thing right?

Yet you're Gov is, having to Inadvertently pay this 'Good Collection Out Again', all back and more as collected tax we gave - you took. Paid in wages - paid now back to pay ((Job-centre staff teams)). The bus journey asked I take.

The moral of my story is, I don't require travel expenses (to reach my destination) at the Job centre plus office when really Interviews conducted I attend. Check ups on my furtherance well being can save (me and you time) via Telephoned, or Online emails/or via Postal service. Interviewed quickly briskly - saving me on travel expenses only to claim them back later.

So claiming back from you (the gov) is pulling money away from government subsidies every time I travel to see you.

But hey, look, not a problem cause Bus companies are loving it, right? You're making any short falls from these guys - tax they give back. And keeping them in high profit - that must good then correct? Nevertheless losing it again, only to pay our dedicated teams at the Jobcentrepluses - along with my forked out Travelling Expenses.

A Voluntary Job in my Village creates the highest Economical best Outcomes. I see no other Logic born Autistic cloth.

Is there no right or wrong answer? Or is it one argument, a conclusion you reach - you're not shifting, your not changing.

Having said all this do you see why A.S. people can't Change to conclusions they reach? One conclusion is given more leeway to breathe.

Asperger's look after their kind, you - your kind.

I'm trying to do the right thing here by you, Authoritarians. Maybe I see logic differently.

You say: problems with Voluntary work, Simon, 'Yes, is helping out Working? Sure, but still is not paying TAX, cause he's not like **Working** for an **Employer direct.**'

Even if Simon Voluntary Works, we are still going to try coaching Simon away, or at least trying to into a FULL TIME WORK Job position, as the ((**End result**)).

So whenever Simon goes for Work-Focused-Interviews, **he's** immediately **expected** to pretend **he's looking** or **Interested** for **Work**, when in-fact my truth is, he looks for work in freedoms, 'he's juiced In.'

Therefore he's always saying: I'll Work Voluntary whilst turncoat to saying yes, I'm looking for (Work still) - yet it is actually furthest root of action, I'll be wanting following as Simon. Many decrees I cried out my explanations.

Work is fine and, if like me, you have served out your college days then Work you're lined up for takes a different root from Simon, the many ways great minds evolve. Simon is skilled in Carpentry. He served his apprenticeship moons ago and is now vindicating he use his skills in freelance alternative suggestions

- Small business - who knows - a place where Simon is left quiet, as long as he's fruitful in his ideas. The practical applications; the productive; the advantages of showing freedom in your Business our/my higher levels respected.

I See a Plaque on the wall once, visiting my friendly Job Centre, (and for most part, it is yes friendly). This Plaque with Crest like feathers around it read:

((We Invest in people)). I only wish I could have pinched it as a reminder - hung on my bathroom's wall.

The uncomfortable natures I am - rendered to your glossy brochure plan, I find it makes me ill. Agreeing to plans 'others' want for me.

So I don't lose benefit I am given another 3 months of limbo. Paralysed in helping the World out of my admissions, My forward Plan. My gifts I come bearing, wondering In a 3 month ball park zone, from when I was last Interviewed each Time.

Justifications I fight 'are my ways' - my appeal losing soul - who I like be. My Gifts are not of 3 Kings, I Serve only 'One.'

Having Asperger's Syndrome, O.C.D, Mental ills thrown my way. Back problems and a Mouth condition called Angina Bullosa Haemorrhagica. A mouth condition where Blood blisters appear, roof, inside cheeks, sides of Tongue, inside mouth.

Even with my many Problems I don't mind gaining Full Employment, I just fear my motivation with my unknown day to day assessment, best Serves Voluntary Sectors where I am less put On. A result Guaranteeing me freer access over my developing body languidness as I come.

Being told the Way I think is almost not allowed, **yet** is **fundamental** with who **I am**, how I grow, show productivity.

You can find weaknesses in my renderings - how I tie a knot, me fighting my own 'Cause' off my own back, against a panel of people who are not A.S. themselves, you easily untie all my knots, re-looping lashing me pushed directions. I respond badly, you may even say Rude. Even when I show willing/kindness is like given the wrong Anaesthetic, strangely I still am Thanking You, which I do.

Feeding a mind with tuned in Rolls Royce Engine Standards, you pass & go my vehicle Mini Club man, I wish not altered. Never lets me open up as I might of liked. The dream in me trodden on. Smiling for your sake, crying inside (knowing this is not me).

Compassionate fake smile I continue cause, it is mandatory to fit In.

Care for you - I do - so wear regardless and smile.

The truth is, I only show function my Internal hands hold my heart's position done my way, less cripples up my Autistic offerings. Don't turn my feet turned In, Wicked Witch of East style, folding in on myself. Then people saying is that guy alright, Cast to my gutter further, a communication broken.

Negative People.

Negative People in my World, I find are our Ones who try Hardest. Negative People gracefully let Positive People win through, fore they shout there is only One True Way, while Negative People will love you no matter Positive no matter Negative, therefore I say he beloved you 2 Ways. The Negative person would Happily run 'Positive', though why Trade in my first Positive Character I like to be, that you said was my Negative.

To be now a Positive Character you mould as what Positive Looks like that isn't me. A Person can be slighted as being a Negative Person, no matter how you try. I find it is Easier to be seen as the many Negatives I am told I am, look down heartened, then there is no expectation of Greatness.

We all should shine emphasis Negative man's Positiveness.

A Negative Man says, let's go the whole hog, knowing

this message is wrong, he carries on regardless, believing now it's (easier to be hated). This is why I believe the many in this World say how can there be a God when so many terrible things plague Us? I respect this as God's Love, no matter of No logic running blue.

Sure you are correct I'd rather he'd not put me through my Trials, though the Way I Interpret God's Love suited on my needs, is how might he know we Love Him, when God Gave Good things Forever Only?

We Receivers of Good things Forever, is in my Tongue explains to You. You Only ever loved God, when he did Good Things for you Forever, when never faulting, when never failing You.

Coming Autistic I tell you I am not sorry. I try where I can treat the many Spectrum's of Positive/Negative people - come as strictly with or with found Interchange respected. Never dismissing (one way) as better one Way look.

I find more Love in Negative People, for they're our camouflaged Positives. Doing a camouflaged Good.

Being Good all the Time - to All People might well make You wonder - am I Loved only because I forever keep Giving, then Giving, then Giving some more? Doesn't Jesus need to perform a Test on his People to See who, when separating the Wheat from the Chaff, who Strayed away and who kept Believing In him, when he didn't Give Us Everything Always?

Does this mean he's vanished from your beliefs he now no longer exists?

Loyalty Good persons know they Owe a debt to Jesus, through any Turmoils we go through, although we can't understand All God's Way, we are not to Question his Ways. Pain Jesus went through on the Cross, Jesus kept praising people, Seeing Only Good of those quick to doubt him, still he breathes Life in his doubters no matter how they mock.

He did as much as could for you. The rest he required something from You.

Try Show him you pull your poured weight entrusted Waters.

Faith doesn't Question, doesn't Serve Others' Questions, cause only a true Sovereign King Questions. No one ever said to Jesus dying, how can there be a God if bad things happen? For Jesus was God. He was among Good and Bad whilst himself dying Cries out amongst battling confusion my lord's Tears.

Non believers and half believers; God is always here keeps giving You that one last Second Chance. How long does he keep holding his hand out without your Full Believe? Do you only believe in God when only logical proves you a Good Worth? Disbelieving exchanged as a believe Science.

Jesus isn't Science he's our History. He is our only One Power above the Law on high. He brought confusion like The Tower of Babel read in Bible.

Lord I don't pretend I understand all your Ways battle of Good and Bad. It less matters I don't understand, I don't Question. I come as a Believer no matter of my confusion cast. God's Test however unfair - had to be this Way I am afraid.

I don't Question our Father, I believe my Fathers guiding presence, for bad in the World you See Is not the makings of my Father.

Bad I see, an Autistic Believer in Christ is only - Satan's heritage, and so when I am asked why would I believe in a World made of Good and Bad things occurring, I can only conclude the Devil is a part of the World's Test while our Father is forever putting Right this Garden of Inhuman.

I just See Good. Walking through I held my Lord's hand; smelling your Fine Robes Father. You asked me first believe Lord, then you Provided still not perfect; though a Test worthy - found your true followers. Shalom Amen.

God struggles he does his best, it is true he cannot Save everyone.

Stop Asking Why? Believing is the Key - I use. Amen.

I Thank God for what he can do, not what he cannot. And I struggle along in guilty gratitude. Made too feel like a King, fore I am just a Servant to my Father. Amen.

Good, living in a World of non believers often I'm looked at oddly sneered at.

Making mistakes in a 'run Positive World', is almost forbidden; it is designer Positive people who'll shine light on a Man's pitfalls.

We have too accept many Negatives and Positives forever running through us, this is how Learning is done - like Car Battery both are terminals Required. Don't Only be One.

I stay Unchanged, I can't reorder my thinking cause it is not politically correct.

God never left me when I myself became this everything that repulsed, a little scarring left, remains stays.

Yet for all God could of done he wrapped his Cloth around me, out stretching his arm, saying! 'this time will you follow me, will you believe me, I offer you love' in a Godless World, so I might test you fairly.

I am preferring aloneness in how I feel. Convincing you of God's existence, is lying to myself, I Believe and that's as far as my Will, extends.

Heavy heartened every battle is fought with a heavy heart. God's love is Hard to reach you fight for God - this is Love. You effort shown Struggle.

You fought thought, people were going to love you a Good ball of energy you. Not true, it is a painful task to shine in Good light.

Choices we make sets apart loyalty.

I live Minority alone.

You will carry on making mistakes no doubt.

Your Religion will leave you at times - no doubt.

The ((Word of God)), will stay with you, ((do not doubt)).

Shalom Amen.

Thinker's outside the box.

Ideally I'm looking for winding down, every 3 month Interviews put to a Stop - something is agreed upon.

Though miss our little Interviews me and Lisa at Havant Job-centre-plus had every 3 months, along with my other kind Advisers over many Years. I should be In the ((Support Group)), not W.r.a.g. Group currently I am In, though who am I to be the judge, of that?

I am not unreasonable guy I come with a PLAN. Something agreed please, which just lately I have found Hope. And Job Centre are Helping me middle of the road, fairness.

Much like taking a Corner on a big 750 cc motorbike, cannot lay rested smooth rides, we all deliberate a safer ride until we're, are on an open stretch.

Working as a **Volunteer**, the safety net remains there for us both.

Working up to 16 hours in W.r.a.g can only be achieved in a Support Group where I am allowed legally earn up to £110ish and keep all my Benefits untouched.

WRAG does claim, you can do all things you can do In a ((Support Group)). Though quoting me on forever unclear changing Information never quite stationary resting In my clear whistles Autistic, Nature.

Government deeming 'help me back into Work', at my age of 41 now 43 - Nearly 44, is more 'uncertainty'.

I said, Lisa my P.A at my last Interview, I request something agreed upon at this Job-centre plus please - that's final, ((lift black clouds - lift)).

It is not I don't love seeing Lisa, my P. Adviser - I do.

I love the way she Smiles back at me - she's one in million, in-fact I feel related, like she's my - Aunty Lisa.

I just want wooden hammer decision reached pleased. Court adjourn rise.

It pains me to bring up often, my conditions in conversation of A.S.

Wishing not come back In Job-centre ever again.

I also need know what Benefits will be affected?

I.e. - ((E.S.A.)), ((D.L.A.)), (Housing benefit & Council Tax).

Looked so many times at Jobs on Internet, in Job-centres. I am just not Interested selling myself outwards, is not In my nature.

Going to Job Interviews they say! 'Aha Aha' - tell me Mr Newell (why do you want this job). I say look I don't want this Job, I am here under restraint - the powers that be. My mind is serviced not your ways. I'm sorry - we will fallout - your job is depressing.

When a person don't like Football or Hockey, there's no point in kitting him out in your badges of honour, he's not interested. I am not Interested.

I have my own Interests obsessive so why would I lie to you?

Asking you only do the right thing, give me back my tools of Interest, before putting your economics first.

There's always Solutions when there is Spirit In man.

Making living World, the only thing worth my while, grabbing my attention is something you care about. Is good grounds, I'll freelance help you.

Uncle Scrooge dropped money, see excitements on the (Christmas faces). A Heart built to Win finds a way prosperity, Shares when your Interest is my Interest. And my Interest is your Interest.

Jobs **holding** an **Interest**, is saying, my blood swims correctness with my family values how your mind Works. I don't waste your Time, Jobs pushed on me.

I hold Interests - yes I do hold them - only in the freedoms left I Educate myself. Doing you Service.

The family man me is not getting there, he's not me.

Show promise wisdoms of your Tax buck, raised in collection to me, most of all to my Cousins in the A.S. Arenas, workers' energy similar. I say that's me energy distributed, money was nothing more than tool of choice, rolling jobs get done, all working relationships completed.

Handed ((golden ticket)) smiling, less struggles - walked me home following is not an easy Ticket we find, living disorderly on Spectrum.

Always a personal element of discorded leasing.

Personally I say - I think you'll always have yourself problems with Asperg people whether they, Working/ Unemployed/or Self employed. They don't mean be Awkward, they just run strong Senses.

You must work with the yeasts of A.S. Productive profit, gave voluntary back.

Working full employment some A.S.s become dominantly pushed into remained responsibility of government property, like cyborg man, universal soldier, Robocop or ED 209. (Isn't right).

Asperger's persons - they go against persons - who systematically day by day, inch away at them. Muscling In on their weakness, turning them the Spectrum disorient round, obeying dominant bully types.

Spectrum disorderlies In full work is this game of inch by inch turning around (an Associate), in any form. 'Spectrum-ed' on the Calender.

Furthermore, I declare shown shaping demanded normal moulds on A.S.s clamping as one doesn't weaken their spring. It only heightens depression, anxiety, bystanders our already overloaded condition.

The Calendars World on Spectra, decision makers far too demanding on a sensitive A.S.'s senses as is.

You want (him/her to Work). More on point you want him yes help out in life. This is not wrong - yet rather than acceptance how he functions, what amazing helpful miracles you would seen from the A.S. not pulled into your lines net, getting quote - so called Jobs done - your way only. Distressed conclusions, minds as fruitful as ours not made a matching pattern.

Instead gave an old story. Seen no repents, in other words. Grey flowers of Authority, which had him slaved into liking you, not one of natural blossom.

Sure he/we smiled - thanked you. Reality reveals his/our hearts fell asleep, rot away. Toll took from him/us.

Even when (powers that be) lighten up in being the fairer Saint these days, motives are still motives same long reach eventual.

Just watered them down hider unclear, not swimming my rungs fair.

Real high sprung Spring of good intention. Run help those (aligned as different) - is a spring uncoiled - your natural shape. Takes you back to your origins no matter unfolded sequences laid.

You cannot seem take away very strict regimes you bound, it is who you are. Continues to set mandates only Grey Ugly duckling.

Searching souls, I found you knew this was wrong, yet your in catch 22, so no I can't blame you. Loyalties you bared sustained Rights.

Passive anger (moves) smoothly undetectable reluctant, still the (lines) of what we see unfair, shows in personas Innocent of fitted In Character. So we humble our self, agree to please, ready to watch lime cemented bricks fall. Work-ability not aligning our Characters - some was only In for Capital gains.

You changed because your thinking came out of Fashion. I remained same Fashion, cause I like Forever Strong.

No changed as A.S. cause we were like witches dunk, batter fry, no dying of swimmers change, you dunk us again, again & again.

William Wallace screaming out, ((Non changer A.S.)) slaved his shackled - this ones coming with us.

Forgiving Aspergs - forgive you. Time after time it's easy think you're right 'we think', when you yourself were led belief correct passage by majority others, so really no blame.

Brain washed under scheme of things, shallows togetherness you once was.

Not caring friends you went with many heights - and found these were not your true friends. They in-fact used you, so serving them you hurt both, (you and us).

Upset hankered friends, lay my best friends inside Tear drops. Sensitivity not forecast. A Grey closed flower forgotten colours; unspoken hurt, believes left heartless. Autistic Outsides show my hidden distress Well Dressed, so you make Instant decisions on what you See. Later you find I am No longer Well Dressed, my Outside is my Inside Cloth.

Fresh Meadows vitalized, smelling colours - ran with loved ones - strong of Independent thinking.

Strong when you give no askance - all my switches controls, A.S.'s free philosophise.

Much energy knocked you down bowling skittles, a heart is not a muscle under Authority, she my heart. Is held up in lost Queues 'little circulate' left leaving A.S.'s distraught.

Less strain more adjustment, is my Home - don't Change.

Open up, loosey goosey.

Asperger's Spectra always try to open kept communication with the World. ((Keep it open,)) set at a frequency he vibrates on, much like a guitar's string resonating at 440hz.

Asking then he work harder than 'this vibration', when already he's showing great promise, better managed work-hard skills. Left to vibrate on his own, in this, his easy frequency, lesser power struggles. Still has (others) forever challenging us, asking us we must fall in line.

On their frequency tied lashed to a mask - that falls, out of Character from us.

Robbing us of our freedom, our identity. Movement is hard, movement is restricted, our kept held of tightly 'before Values' is items of now re shelved, re-branded. Heinz Oxtail tin soups we credited ourselves on before, is nothing more than labels ripped from us thrown to the floor sheep shearing without care. Like a Sergeant demoted to Corporal for a new Company is in town under Captain red neck hot head. A new order on pallet, arrives - sweeping away old labels. Precious time A.S.s paid in is now pure Industrial waste. Relabelling Starts here.

Presentation, good working relations (hold) - yet for how long this time? Long enough my memory traces back A.S.s old empire traditional values. Long enough Captain red neck stays friendly - or does he flare up unequivocally? Bringing the best of my A.S. awkwardness - singing him a tune.

Determined (never to let go) is A.S. truth, like your carrying a Million squid in a satchel, crossing enemy invested jungles, looking to find untainted Waters.

The way (your Normal Jungle Animal friends) on their frequencies, 'wants you' echoing the same Animal calls of the wild. Tainted or untainted matters not, (a condition born of development) can't change. Shouldn't change.

The Kookaburra, for instance, of Native Australia sitting in his old gum tree - echoes.

Hello: Asperger's. Asperger's. Asperger's.

The way your (any) normal frequencies - (common to you), is working hard (forever dominates), your person category, to see known others pull their weights, detangles, Works. Although A.S. show you awareness, understands how (you) must Operate. The A.S himself in his own known frequency vibration Category, just Sees you shouting anger, hot-headiness on your part. However the A.S. Sees in Others, from his own closest Category resembling, a formations that he's Categorized, is by showing 'Separation' so no dominance within our own Wavelength, a fight to stay looking different - cause we Are.

The A.S. tries to show things as easy, not to panic you, with side effects (others) not on the Spectrum, (see as weak). Our Quietened mind used in progress.

Hard-work (progressing), correct adapted ticket, yes it is. Bullying hard work is not friendly. Hard-working frameworks of you and us, is! motivation breeding excitement help towards the Jobs, done in life quicker you 'were allowed' develop. Take flight of Difference.

Working hard saying demanding you think like a Neuro-typical only is reluctant, allows our mind no development. The A.S. forever Survives in a one Conditional juice so Sees (workable Growth) produced via heart and soul relaxed hard work only.

Asperger persons 'want/share' that, when they do. (They are hushed up), immediately cut off.

You want us involved, become part of a work hard society in one message - we smile say sure just leave out control, devised energy. Work our interests, we'll work yours and we will share as (Moderates). A.S.s can adapt - though fundamentals don't change.

Unsettling noises make our nerves bad, more so than ((N.T.s)), so wherever possible limit unwanted noises. Limit jokes, limit work banter. This is idleness to the hard work message, you first asked of us.

Have consideration over the noises you make please, pleasant noises, 'happy voices not a problem'.

Just distractions, unnecessary noises Asperg shuts down - (freezing him on this spot), able to move not.

Then if more serious 'goes into Meltdown.'

An A.S.'s message is clear then, yes?

Don't take from him - though do give, the way A.S. has, shall give freely.

Talk gently he has only small ears hearing, breathing in through his ears, like opening eyes of a baby just born, (must develop), this hearing cared for.

Not just when you feel like doing your good bit, but when you (stay with him), so convincing him into confidence.

(Don't stay with our cousin A.S.) off guarding him, breaking his nerves this is not working hard. It's working wrong. Random people forever up and down - doesn't give confidence back to our A.S., the A.S. I am.

Drawing to a close.

Well I hope you got something from my 2nd book, we've covered as before a lot of ground, I barely have started - so stay or rest a book Marker here.

Join me in my 3rd Book, strength in me prevail. My main Aims now heads towards back to further Education, University since Writing Full time on Benefits is considered not helping You Out.

Going back to University, I've chosen to gather Information studying at: University of Surrey. The University of Surrey is in Top 10 best Universities in United Kingdom, and has won a 1st Place Category best University found 'Graduates', Employ-ability Employment within 6 Months. It does come at a Cost from my Prospectus 2016 I read from, £9000 Student Fees each year.

Though there are Ways through this, that all will take me much consideration.

I can apply government loan, and you pay back only after

Graduation when in Employment and earning over £21,000 annually of 2016's date. Which sounded almost too good to be true, so I'll look into this later.

There were many enticing Other Ways to negotiate £9,000 Student Fees I quickly read, in my Prospectus. You can be paid by an (Employer) a Salary on Professional Training Placements, or at least negotiating some other Worked plan forward, reducing your Fees from what was quickly read. Though at my age 43, I'm not any Employer's long Solution. My physical body not so strong these days.

My Mental agility is a Tap Dancer, I just wish both physical and mental connected my joining. Enthusiasm is my bags of Mental state, my physical state is clumsy awkward, dealings laid with my Others. This is why I'm looking hard, I want to find Employment after sitting my A Levels, and perhaps studying at my chosen University or College, embarking on say a Solo career as Guitarist, or in a Jazz ensemble Quartet. People I can entrust around playing in late Night Smokey bars. Restaurants. Clubs. Hotels. Theatre Opera Orchestral Accompaniment. And so on. Many Avenues reviewing.

I can also try Volunteer - gain experience with, a Jazz or Blues band 'willing' kind enough to take me on under their Wing whist Studying, slow turning me over into their Payroll, so I might make a Living. The many Weathers we fight On. My Benefits, then can Stop, though rather than abandon me, it should be Noted I'm Autistic, and can lose Employment as fast as I find Employment.

So Safety Nets should unroll help all vulnerable Claimants at Jobcentres, as they an Organization themselves - with a Job they're paid to do. Should keep Encyclopedia size Log books, where finding a Band to Join, isn't uncommon place. When I say, my last Band didn't work out, what Band choice and style genres of Music may I find, join residency willing to Employ me Today at Job Centre.

Claiming Benefit Money isn't my first choice, when I find I am at Odds with Others a Job centres Job. Should keep narrowing in my Target Information, so I myself am more likely stay In long Employment Once my Interests all persons Interests remain continue Customizing. Don't Stop Tailoring, don't settle 2nd best, you said you're Worth more. Job Centre and your New Employer, should never lose contact, even whilst I am (free) of Benefits. Any new Company, Org, Corporation, Industry you join hands employed Employment. They should say you're the Boss. I make you make the Decisions. I take responsibility, watch my Company meet Profit Targets.

Being employed has never been so much Fun, so let us carry on Opening doors. After all it is what you said you wanted, so I am here at your Request.

Paying Student fees of £9,000 at Universities. There were also, I see, Special Support Grants available if you qualify as having certain Disabilities, which I 'don't'. I have certain (Conditions) as Autistic, so not sure how all this will fare out. More Importantly though than All this, I must gain - Typical Entry requirements to study as an Undergraduate, so in my case, I want to study Music, so requires 3 A levels Graded A-B-B must Achieve. I look at Grade 8 level Music.

A break away from my over active Asperg mind calls, walking myself down, backing away to Asperg free territory, took relief.

Home with a simpler Simon, low functioning. Deconstructed to simpler forms, back to unlearning (empty dinner plate), listening to Beethoven (Ludwig Van).

Karma strolling with friends, my war paint washed out.

Pulling on quiet Memories I recline.

The Tug of War, I shall carry out life my way.

And you opposing, if opposing. We must pull in all directions on your fashion wheels. Uneasy yet understanding, perhaps.

Us tugging hard this way now the A.S. Community is drawn on strengths new, powers fought laid down.

Exchanging Battle-shields - defence won our Sunnier tomorrow, digging In A.S. muddy boots.

This game Tug war ((Over)).

Hopes not see new generations, history followed as Autism/Asperger's reliving far to out suffered. Ignorance little known of them, living on Calendar struggles.

A question of I do for you, you do for me, is not a question!

Not always a question - what you say, you can do for us the Autistic?

Allowance what we say, (we can do for you). Flower opening stem cells once rejected of your heart's garden, sharing ideas in Sunny game of life.

Many normal people In life - just moan.

Asperger's don't really care bout all that, just forever Happy.

Triumphed against his Sea of troubles, smiling when hard is - hard Yes.

I suffer within Mild Asperger's as One with me main embodiment shadowing.

I have Mental ills, lessened when Conquer Conker my Way threaded on my shoelace I smash over come.

A bag of future/hope.

Sir, all very well giving disabled people futures hope, the all much familiar 'your Visions' in the Marketing, you heard me run through. Copy catted tongued as Civil Servant attitudes take affects on those not born of such laws ridiculous, yet distributed non the less, since we all are strangers of Good and Bad seen.

We of many Disorders found we already made our minds up (fights gone over), not in greedy in maintaining a - One Vision approach.

Only we see our best fitted footed future forwards, one

bead on at one time leisured.

Muscling in slowly turning keys, naive people don't know - they have been 'are being had.'

Forced live your Visions we do, yet less work still achieved, more of same sameness dished up one lump or two. Those you made follow you not given choice, was seen from us, 'over bearing you'.

I hurt your feelings I see, you did me too, run a mile for me - my intentions are good. Sung Blues.

Narrowing my Arrows short sleeves, pulled tight, taught tension - braved of teeth. I cleverly turned short skirt, my Welsh Kilt, my life around your handkerchief - Sir.

Original Karate Kid.

Karate Kids, (cocky confidence) is played by Ralph Macchio. **Daniel LaRusso.**

Got Daniel L - (in trouble, a lot) in these, the films Karate Kid. (I. II. III).

The same (cocky confidence) Ralph Macchio mentions, in an audience Interview I watched online, had me summarizing 'good comparisons' our own cousins In Asperger Syndrome we find ourselves.

Daniel is my (close resemblance), bubbling volcanic hot waters (time time, & again), I as one A.S. distribute my familiarities born scenes witnessed throughout, Karate Kids adventures with close ally friend - Mr Miyagi.

So us with our Asperger's you will see the **Daniel LaRusso** in us. Our character we wouldn't swap for all remembered, China Tea.

This **Cockiness Daniel** puts over is the Asperger's **Rudeness**, 'you see, same in us'. I best describe this Rude/Cockiness like this! - what I call - dub:

Mediterranean / **co**cky / **ru**de / **ch**ild / **co**nfidence:

Many people still to this day, **unfortunately**, take the

wrong way attitudes, seen in younger people more so, though living just as strongly in elders.

My, Self dubbed diagnosis is dubbed: Med / cocky / rude / child / confidence.

Abbrev: (M.c.r.c.c).

My M.c.r.c.c. (Initialism or acronym), thing going on gives you my indications word for word: ((5 words - in-fact)) - Daniel with A.S.s, Share.

Mediterranean is (**word 1**) meaning= both Daniel/A.S.s live in a Mediterranean naivety World.

Cocky is (**word 2**) meaning= both Daniel/A.S can't help their own emulating body talk they see as harmless. Normals not like us, see as an Insult.

Rude is (**word 3**) meaning= both Daniel/A.S.s play out a Rudeness **Others** See in them **as, offensive.** That we believe, is our: 'holiday Mediterranean Aura

Charms' hence - knocked often, deep in brokered feelings we felt is, Normal comfort natural born in, of us.

Child is (**word 4**) meaning= both Daniel/A.S.s no matter of adult grown up language, we became, through the years inheritance remains unchanged. Our returning home keys brought back. (Our child behaviours) therefore a comfort blanket world we yearn, people caring. Returned home through complicated (mazes), to simpler forms, where love was always abundant and memory was less clouded.

Confidence is (**word 5**) meaning= both Daniel/A.S.s exude confidence, his World asks for. Yet knocked the confidence - we banged. Big steel drums. Thumping in us then left, broken.

It is true to say the Character Daniel in Karate Kid films, 'did not' have A.S. or Autism. Yet it gives you some scope, diversities in which both N.T.s and A.S.s, crossover in likenesses found. And yet still very separate.

To whom qualifies Normal, whom qualifies A.S., is nothing more than a see-saw affect, effect.

Daniel was from my perspective at least, borderlines A.S., meaning his own language is stuck in paralysis, he's frozen. He didn't function in Normal cause he's a different Normal to Normal. And he'd not function qualified in A.S. cause he'd be (pond hoping) back to Normal. Finding, no comfortable zones.

Often you are strictly A.S or you are strictly Normal. Peoples minds I've, observed find no, - In-between.

So an A.S. Person with added Normal characteristics can, pond hop in (both life's) and when told his Normal, they forget (the A.S is), aligned closer to his own alliance of A.S. Simply because generally he does unfold as A.S. resemblance, in most things he's challenged the tasked Signatures A.S. Hand-prints. Through seen dis-likeness or disgust certain Normals gives back as, obvious dislike.

We learned/trained to separate ourselves, from (them who say), **I just** don't **like him.** With no reasoning just (don't Like him) and why perhaps A.S.'s forever go it Alone.

Karate Kid was a film of the 80's, you should be familiar with.

Daniel LaRusso would use some might say termed as (sarcastic lines) in Movie and during the film. Cocky Confidence defiant Daniel like Asperger Syndromes (we're this). The same - unashamed.

Same in regards, our confidence - is beautiful Hong Kong. Yet what feels pleasant to us is seen as Vietnam in us wherever we display our rested coins on table. We thought fought A.S. was beautiful what was right in us, Cocky C is apparently wrong. And why many A.S.s suffer with their nerves, more so than said Normals. Harmless Cocky C, I emulate is make-up, apart my Character.

We thought this way ((our A.S., Ways)) was Natural, so we call our A.S. (our Normal).

Defined frameworks, coding us as - diagnosed symptomatic s. Leaning we are, by natural birth. So diagnosis's found, every single day **transformed** some **said normals** (later), found carrying A.S. philosophies.

Cocky C, is what we are naturally, though is glared at through the Nostrils often. Good cockiness not aimed at you. Our way of showing love joining In, we'd hope (was me - In you, with you).

We never ourselves, never, take people the wrong way, baffled by the evil stares of, given peers.

So why asked in earnest, (the/they, other people), take us all the wrong way, throwing discomfort blanketed everywhere we walk, they walk - I walk.

Breaking us more so, (in hurt we hurt already), no other time.

We are open as A.S persons cause we are broken in (our preferred Private), so we come out our comfort zone, in the what we believed, (you wanted of us). Bashed knocked (open or private), we are condemned in pleasing you, as are we condemned in not thinking as you, do. Nor does it feel right.

We tie our rope around, our tent pegs differently.

Is, - (as we - tackle/do - our jobs), such a bad thing?

Those who know you (don't require you watch, every single word you say). Though to strangers, this battle continues forever expanding in Loop-de-loops.

We need a Cocky freedom I am afraid so to test, - can we really be ourselves, and still be loved?

Sure we can watch our, Step, (**often we do**) though sorry I say we, hold against you, for chaining us **to** be **this**, (forever careful, around you - guy I am).

I do express reach out saying, asking, don't padlock my expressive freedoms for although (A.S. I am) my character is different to other A.S.s, no doubt.

In same tone, 2 Normal persons are categorized, (Normals) - again no doubt, their 2 Characters, (are possibly different) so you have an interchange within people going on, unresolved debates to whom, is - Right.

A different footed animal we Aspergs line our: purple silk inner jackets (A.S. defined), is not a reason to now make disassociation.

Using - good energy is hard, so no dropping your guard being like all the rest easier followed like, (Joe blow) Normal is easy.

Takes effort/struggling, not to deny, a once good energy lost art we hoped. (Real you), inside you.Many suffer out cry, Designer Human Emotion, routines.

Strangely reassured, people with a Conditional **disorder** are tossed quickly over as (**Normal**), so when they do quote (function well) yet set conditions on their disorder remain (forgotten in transit) by and large, by the many.

It is then, people of our **Conditioning** requires become (the rendered Useless), laughing stocks, by strong dominant Normals.

Just so you know (Asperger's '**is-a**' Condition) of what each A.S. person requires. Asperger's is not necessarily a (disability) at all.

A.S. is focused as: a **disorder** more so, to how he functions in the Normal World.

Asperger's Syndrome eternally is challenged using such deemed (cocky confidences) Ralph as **Daniel LaRusso** was challenged. Reminding familiarities bore of my own Condition. No matter the designs of D.N.A you attach as you, we all, **Normal** or **A.S.** broker as. (One or the other), and so we hurt just like the same.

The way A.S make connections with Normal persons (**and vice** that **versa**), is largely dependent factors...? Are we both **friendly** happy characters.

If you answered, Yes. Then Normality - is shared and founded.

Again Spectrum calendars - (often back down), wondering what have deserved done wrong... conditioned different.

We can't understand why Others are not taking to Us,

for this is genuinely how always expressed ourselves. Amongst our own diagnosed Persons or as a family regulated Normal.

People say - ((**be yourself**, who else **can you be**)), when you are!, you're knocked for it scattered.

Hitting the hive for honey trickling, we just wanted to be ourselves honey smelling tasting A.S. orientated.

No hiccups though, is never a place granting promise I show full confidence. Poetic rhythms, awkward stagnated. Awkward rhymes, help us remember. Reasons I am free.

Have you ever noticed Way - **some people say:**

'**See you Later**', like you owe them something, or are indebted to their every word. On tender hooks till you meet them next, is no way to carry on.

Well - we, (as we Are), walk not this feeling of a **contract** between **people**, you must abide or else. Sure you must stay in check, but not enough that it's making you ill with worry. The A.S. **by-passes this control.** We accept you belong obliged to others yes, you got to work with people sure.

Yet **don't agree** with it.

Don't agree with them.

We after we walked passed these kind of people, very loosely unbutton (both left/right - shirt cuffs), so **to stay** who we're **freedom.**

Bill Furlong.

Bill Furlong has Autism and Author of 2 books currently: (Where there's a Bill there's a Way) and (Bill's Way).

Bill himself, suffers affects his diagnosis presents to him. Autism I believe. His condition takes stronger sufferance of my own condition under Asperger's. Though to me he's just Bill, very Normal in every way.

Reading Bill's first book, it made me cry inside, I sympathized with my light strain Mild Asperger's.

Me and Bill are friends on Computer's social media. Having read Bill's first book (and liking it), humanistic. I decided to search out Bill on facebook one day. Sent a friend request, thought nothing else of it.

It had been some year or so, longer possibly. When a red sign caught my attention on face-book, it was my friend Bill. He had accepted my friends request.

I heard through the grape vine our friend Bill had published his 2nd book.

I cannot remember details to the points of accuracy, who made my awareness known Bills 2nd book, was now out there. Just remember I was so pleased he got recognition he deserves. Awareness to his condition told by someone, genuine.

I rarely if ever talk too Bill on the computer. Nevertheless, backs of my mind, I made a reservation to grab a copy of Bills 2nd book. I heard was available.

I wasn't given no clues how I might obtain this 2nd follow on book Bill worked hard on. So after looking briefly myself on internet and phoning around the various bookshops in Portsmouth. I made no leads in possessing Bill's book.

Involved in my own 2nd Book Manuscripts my attention span, had no time to slow down. So I detracted until time was more my friend.

I posted an article on face-book once - I was astounded, Bill made a comment.

I accepted Bill's comments... and since he contacted me, I took opportunity.

Opportunity, asking him politely, how I might go about grabbing his 2nd book called: Bill's Way.

Bill was very nice towards me, and he informed me I could grab the 2 copies I was after. Either via direct at his home address. Or he said Simon, my book is available at - ((Black Stones)).

I searched the Internet once again. To find (Black-

Stones) didn't exist in Portsmouth. I could only speculate Bill had got it wrong and so I made an enquiry instead at (**Water stones** bookshops). I still had no joy.

Black Stones bookshop was rolling in my mind, I eliminated Water Stones.

I then remembered how when coming home from my own publishers at Tricorn Books. A Bookshop - close to (Tricorn Books) did exist.

However, this bookshop was called ((**Blackwell's**)), so after making my own investigations.

I got back to Bill almost immediately. He admitted he had got his wires crossed wrong, and apologized.

Yes **Blackwell's** Bookshop was where I'd find my 2 copies. I was excited. I told Bill I'll catch the train from my home County of Surrey into Portsmouth, via train methods.

Cost me £14 to £21 on Train Return Tickets. I arrived at: Portsmouth **Blackwell's** bookshop.

I was devastated, the damn bookshop was closed. Are you kidding me. I was peed off to say the least, the very least.

So I thought stuff it, and grabbed a - **Subway** 6inch meal. Stuffed my face - making me happy.

I had only arrived on (**Good Friday**) back last Easter gone 2015, of all days. So my journey was one of a wasted one.

I went home back to Surrey. I was busy decorating my flat.. so I continued on.

My daughter Natasha was feeling down - a few weeks later... so I took it upon myself. Take the Train, and quickly dropped in a Card of sympathies. The hostel she currently resides.

I eradicated two birds with one stone my second visit back into Portsmouth. And so took a slow walk to Blackwell's also. Once again walking through Guildhall

Square. Past Queen Victoria. I arrived at Blackwell's. ((Now **Open**)).

The man in bookshop was rather camp. So I joined in and gave him my camp side. I said do you keep in stock a book named (Bill's Way). He walked with me stretched up, and took the last 2 copies off the shelf.

We must of chatted 30 to 40 minutes, before I made my purchase. I managed too get away from my camp friend. I walked straight out of Blackwell's, making headway back to Surrey thinking gee whiz, what a lovely fellow.

The camp guy.

My Mum came to visit me a few weeks later and still in the brown paper bag, was Bill's book. I was so pleased to say my friend Bill, had his 2nd publishing.

My Mum was happy - I kept her up-to date with Bill's new release.

I felt Bill's 2nd book played into his strengths rather than his weaknesses. To me at least I see a different side to Bill from his first standards, raised his game pitch.

Bill made a point in his 2nd book page 110.

Suggestive felt a disconnection with me. Preference autobiographical.

He stated Simon's 1st book was more of a collection of continual arguments and statements rather than his preference. Autobiographical.

Which I cannot disagree pretty much that was True.

He says Simon's 1st book warnings you may disagree with his own political stance. I am glad Bill shared.

I took responsible measures declaring my own failings to my readers. I am a newbie to book Writing. I made as stated no qualms why I approached my 1st book without so much as a dustpan and brush effect. I always present my first self tatty. My good works come once scoped a lesser person. This is an Autistic way I adapt.

Scrambled messages A.Syndrome bares on me - runs you low functioning A.S. I am. I am broken too perform Greatness forever. Until loved Low and High functioning.

You may always freely disagree with me. I am not here with Change you. Just please remember I am Different (when disagreeing).

Honestly I just want to be liked/loved as a low key fun authenticity side too me. So most A.S.s play down their high - functionalities.

I was aware my first book was a hard hard read. My only intention was to inform my readers if you thought my first book was hard reading, as my low functioning self (image if you will), uncomfortable feelings (I gave you reading). Triple my 1st books uncomfortable passages. You're coming closer now with the struggles many A.S.s are met with every **single** day.

Good works, it's duly aligned to how much my A.S. Cares, they want you to love them as failures, and successes in equal measuring. I know I can be both, and find no progression just as the Successful A.S. There's more in my friendship than surrounded in successful only.

I help people by not shining too brightly and so when we tame our high functioning self, we are moaned at again for having (fun in failure). We were hated as successful A.S.s, we were hated as failures. Where does 'like and love' survive knowing this? Well to be liked and loved, you must show others Failure and Success (hold hands).

We generally enjoy the escapism it offers for always (one, or the other) brings, two narratives brought along Ripe and rotten fruit. (The balance).

So look we are fighters for likes loved in, only (two) possible arenas.

To be the best, you should accept you should Care, maintenance regulates both alive.

Bill made clear, his best thing about my 1st book. He explained, was a message on last page (paying homage to Bill Furlong).

The Author Simon said himself, just how much he had enjoyed my book.

Bill's 1st book was good read. Though like me it is my own, believe. Bill showed (high functioning Bill), in book 2 - Bill's Way. More so.

In-fact... I'd go as far too say, I prefer reading novice Authors. I feel more love. Without built Credentials on demand.

My Homage paid with Bill's book, wasn't just his 1st book alone. I gave him respect (in both books), cause I am a nice guy, cause they were top-notch.

I like Bill's style of Writing. He brings something new to the table.

I don't require (Autobiographical), in my own essence Authors walk that's Bill's way. And why I love difference.

I work my audience of readers intention crowbar in difference.

I know me and Bill are on the Spectrum. We remain good friends.

I hope I meet for a pint with Bill soon. Not too iron out our differences cause I like Bill just way he is. That is why I paid Homage to Bill.

I was only aware of Bill Furlong - when Gail my friend and publisher gifted me with Bill's Book. *Where there's a Bill there's a Way*.

Chapter 20.

Good News. I may, Work towards, Self-employment. Small business venture.

Hooray, lights glimmer options absolution.

Finally (option flags) of my future, in my palms.

I use a (well versed expression) such as (futures in, palms of my hands) - lightly brushed on, hardly traced.

Still - this far In, best solution to my problems. I'll explain shortly.

Complete control over my handling, within all things 'my life'. Dream (past) not making my horizon, before offered.

It is true to say my **3** to **5** monthly, **W**ork **F**ocused **Interviews continues...** so handing me back - responsibility, faithfulness, entrust to just how you say 'get on with it' backing, governing bodies entities, remains (monitored).

Here is a little talk, one such Interviews conducted, me and Lisa at Job-centre plus office, were discussing one time.

My best breakthrough this far, within, future Date.

I say a (little talk) - though I tend run into (1 hour up say - 1 hour 20 minutes.)

One thing discussion led eclipsed to another. And this is when Lisa my P.A. said Simon, with a pause... why don't you go into **SMALL BUS**INESS.

I beamed Lisa my famous Smile.

Work-focused-Interview with P.A Lisa from Hayling Island

Ports, conducted At: 15:35 hours: 26th June 2014.

Dread, Work-focused-Interviews, as difficult say, what you want. The odds lay stacked in their favour they control certain society's strings. Or so I thought!

Today 1st time in ages... I felt we made some headway.

I love Lisa my Personal adviser - no not like that, she's married damn you, you know like helpfulness wise.

What we discuss is private between us - and that is how it stays.

I was before attending my Interview on this one day, preparing what Jobs as a 'Sufferer on the Spectrum' (I could do) - either Voluntary my preferred route correct course of antibiotics. Or a said choice into full-time Work, preferred option it is thought, Government and Taxpayers voted Allegiance. And mine if only Flexible Work was an option Smiling.

Self Employment ventures is good Grounds I can also Angle. In within my 'Options'.

I keep narrowing a better Autistic Choice. And Thanked Lisa.

65 Stop.

I highlight my own taxpaying alignments. A Job requiring, turn up each day and Tax - is paid. What of those who work-harder in ((alternative ways)) who can't pay Tax? up-to day you reach 65 retirement age... and rising.

Oh you cannot retire at 65 nowadays you say.

Especially 2020 on-wards I hear reverted. Where might looking forward once magic Islands ((of 65)) security trod solid. Goal our ancestors fought a looking forwarding too. And Working Hard with knowing there's a Bridge Closer waiting to Greet Us, called 65.

Retiring at 65 means just that In my mind. For a platform in life... (must rest).

If he decides he can work on... unaided, happy by laws dominating him all his past life gone, it is at this (magic age) you earned a ticket to do many things more your way - surely.

People living longer is an awful bedrock excusing why retirement age is rising rising. There are always better Answers that leaves (65, where Traditionally), it is felt best Strong.

Rules of 65 were set in, (stone). Not to be tampered, majority our traditional ancestors wrote these laws. It is the golden rule... we all meet a deadline look forward.

Take this **rule away**, (what we have), 'we have no Island where rest' only water upon vast water. With no stops in place.

Personally I hold believes making people work beyond 65 is ludicrous. This is their time in life, this is governments thanking each individual, Service they provided. So now in respect in return, governance helps you (into a lesser paced life). Still Working of course, yet your way - without all the laws.

Work you do - as hobbies, for exampling.

Giving unbounded. Donating Tax in less formal agreements.

Hobbies; Balsa-wood planes. Boats Model Yacht's you Sell from no pressuring.

Working with (65) in mind is Man's goal Aim. One works towards.

(You, take this away), you see nothing but big oceans paddling Ores deep in - forever water.

Everyone must reach a certain home-base. And so for me 65 is this home-base we see horizon.

Hobbies at retirement, take on all the things you couldn't do - when you, were Working. And why retiring at 65... is key, to not breaking your dreams.

You kept held dear.

A Special day is Retiring. Crossing new borders. Home safe.

A Holiday you saved for, (shouldn't be cancelled). Nor should your retirement.

Many persons' in life are not principled In such large huge amounts of Time, deducted of 65's Original plan. Living longer equates 'you did so, because', you retired near 65'. Not 70.

A free land, free country, Works hard till I tell you, I must rest. It is a free Country, (only it isn't - you cannot).

Denied options, (free Country). Working voluntary manners producing same to bettered results. Health rewards in free Country. No stigmas attached.

You live with factoring your never be rich. Just principled.

Just happy.

Explain again.

Back at Job Centre, discussing my options, we went from me 'taking a Voluntary Job', in my Community as a **Dog Walker** to a Cat feeder, around old peoples Homes.

I also had taken, a long list of **18 Jobs**. I said I could do as a preferred Voluntary option.

I recently attended a Work Focused Interview on: 2nd Oct 2015.

I moved to Surrey from Portsmouth. Hampshire. Jan 2015.

Lisa is not my P.A. any more. Although she remains history's door when Checking up, is called upon. Example, checking my ACTION PLAN with vital information relied upon - as gospel.

Guildford is my new Job-centre plus. Woodbridge Rd.

My new Personal adviser is ((Imelda)) an Indian lady I believe very gracious.

And more recently ((Sally)), my favourite P.A.

I attended my Work-focus-Interview at 13:00hrs on 2nd Oct 15.

The security guard signed me in. He was especially nice toward me today they usually can show bolshie.

Imelda my new P.A., checked my ACTION PLAN from past history stated on her computer. Then she ran me off a copy.

I got home and hovered over my ACTION PLAN. It concluded... in one small area, that an Interview conducted on 19. 06. 2013 - just brief example this extensive ACTION PLAN laid, 'the following'.

His Mum continually answered for Simon with an explanation mark attached, like this !

I wasn't sure how I should take this, !

Was this wrong... or right... I just did not know?

What I do know however, Is my Mum is there for me, and or my Step father Paul. Always. (At times, make possible).

They understand my condition my Mum and Paul do. Know care enough. They defend a broken voice in me I (locks). I Author Better 'not without a Pen' just left Alone.

Explain ((my condition)), my own emptiness I feel supports best, talked with supported larger groups the Author of natural human I am not.

Misunderstanding heard from ((my voice only)) is easy washed over. And why my Mum and Paul, often spoke a better heard message open communication I lack.

It is only a book I Write clearly because I am left Alone.

Vulnerability to come across as Normal... I do. In job-centres-offices.

Manoeuvre an opening upon me - 'is both', mentally damaging in my short and long runs. Agreeing to All.

When crept cracks of A.S... ((display normal)), as my temporary tension. Means I start off well with people giving them their Normal - they ask for.

Any Normal taken from me. Rotates back, with Asperger's Syndrome my Natural back lights.

Again, I am wondering why - (I'm losing friends) people angry... changing face of A.S., that don't change.

Putting me in places, I come across **Normal** randomly only lasts, in the short nicely conducted Interviews. Peoples whose job outer of my world live, (strong Normal lives). Cannot hear a rhetorical Spring the A.S turns, when challenged. And perhaps why my career path Sings not from, let us share the same Hymn sheet.

My Work-focused-Interview on 2nd Oct 15 at 13:00hrs went reasonably well.

I discussed I am locked in my Saddle writing, my 2nd book.

I told her I tried 2 weeks of Voluntary ((Bell-ringing)), in my Village. I very much enjoyed. However, I felt obliged my weak mind Autistic go down pub with my fellow bell-ringers, and was split Autistic. I would of been fine Socially Interacting with my fellow bell-ringers, I am sure - Kind people.

And Edward was Autistic another fellow bell-ringer I met along the way.

I lose my strict mind Interacting and am vulnerable to Normal I present myself as, Imagery first casts. Therefore, as much I enjoy getting Out and About, I tend not to offer too much, Friendship. My idea was do my voluntary work go home. With no Social involvement.

I just didn't wish lose my focus. (This volt job campanology - is/was, an Outlet only). My main attraction must effort In Authoring. Writer of Books.

I'd like later try Bell Ringing again if and when time

allows.

I discussed also with my new Personal Adviser Imelda, I'll compensate my (book writing) with, volunteering work (down on the Farm). In around my surrounding Village. One such, (Volt job).

Under took considerations, I shall make enquiries (Farm Work), later on book finishes.

As is usual much was discussed in my Job-centre-Interview.

I discussed (**self employment**) as my root Interest. Next time I shall mention going back to College/Uni with a view Full-employment. An Employer understanding, prepared Invest In myself focused healthy happy. The Way I come.

I discussed taking a College course in (Copy Editing and Proof Reading) as a future plan perhaps. Leaving options open, I thanked Imelda (P.A.) and shook her hand.

She then drafted me up **my next:** Work Focused Interview for:

18th March 2016 at 13:00hrs.

I said Imelda my P.A., I should have my book finished, by this time.

My books completion, I'll revert draw up plans, portfolios, business templates, business forecasts I propose at my, next Interviews.

Regarding Self-employment with Job-centre teams.

Whilst liaising with Enterprise First.

((**Enterprise First**)) is an Organisation helping people into business. They work in close proximity currently liaising with (Job Centre plus).

Or I instead, take root College study my A Levels; with Uni in mind or a College best adapted my Music leanings.

Or just Subjects my new mind swings.

Carrying a (jobs short list) in rucksack and walking with.

Throw your Glasses on Simon your Job-centres that way.

Jobs from considerations carried, - some went out box - ideas like:

1. Deep Sea Fisherman.

2. Leaflet dis rib.

3. Making Piggy banks out paper mache from old Manuscript papers hanging around: used notes; dictations; loose paperwork from books 1 and 2. Old DWP Letters what have you. All-sorts of written materials no longer of Importance served used in makings of: (Asperger Ready for Battle books - 1 and 2).

Green Recyclable friendly using creative powers whilst making profit handed over as charity or a tax. Paying revenue considered relaxing laws way tax is rounded up. I pay in piggy banks made.

Making Piggy banks paper mache history laid in rest - Smile.

I'll take Orders customers showing me enthusiastic Interest discussing my go ahead s with my local Job centre.

Simon's self-employment, job Idea's.

New **Self employment** Job direction Options in the wings, Simon you may fight through.

Thanks to Lisa (my last, previous) Personal Adviser... she had introduced me to an Organization called **Enterprise First.** Specializing Support helps people persons' wishing, **Start up small business** Ventures.

Over the Moon, ((I can contribute)) in my World as seen fair by the Taxpayer for '1st **time**', in a long while. Although Self-employment is Risky game so I may drop the Idea like lead weight. And just plug for A Levels/GCSE instead a root into:

1. Musicianship - 2. Politics - 3. Book Writer Author.

Above 3 Career choices I'd happily, Career. And with diverse GCSE and A Levels I Study. I can widen my scope other Careers I fancy.

Again, at my age 43 with problems Autistic residing my Nature, an Employer wants his best from Bunch. So Employ-ability shall require, 'I come different'.

I, in my **New business** may work out a business plan, forging a template (plan of action)… forecasting my directions.

I will Sell '**Guitar Aids**' helping improve the Life of Guitarists.

Normal/Aspergic - Men/Woman, in Projects I Craft.

All my attached problems work best (unburdened). From suffering with a condition called: Angina Bullosa haemorrhagica. Abbrev (**ABH**).

No not that kind of A.b.h.

Is a medical condition. I mentioned earlier! blisters inside mouth. Rupturing brought on by: eating hard crispy foods; under stress; feeling down.

With careful eye, precision. I roll out my Projects, in my new business ventures endured, such as:

Guitar Coffee Tables. - Miniature Fret-boards.

Also Project called: ((Circle of - 5ths & 4ths)) plaques all sizes designs on spec.

(The Circle of - 5ths & 4ths) is a (Circle) a (Clock Face) those who don't know about Guitar. That helps a Guitarist **cycle** through **Key Changes** as one exampling, shows things like a **Keys: Relative Keys...** that's both **Major** & **Minor** - Relatives.

Put bluntly it is very handy. The Circle of 5ths is. And so it's not really something you see too many of on Market. Which is the great shame, and where I step In.

Guitarists can buy these **Circle** of **5ths - 4ths** found most is usual, in diagrams illustrated fantastic-s, inside books bending back books, photo-copying ruined easily, falling flat, every time a door is opened.

So this is a Market as you say: I'd corner - (diagrams crafted into plaques). Without too much Market Research, I know a sharp **corner** is in this **Market,** so cease opportunity within reach.

Other **Projects:**

I am cooking up swimming introduction (as when my Business grows) - are as follows:

Writing Books on: Asperger's Autism Spectrum.

Writing Books on: **Acoustic** and **Electric** Guitar.

Helping focus **Asperger** Orientations as my first fold.

Guitar help - (Beginners to Intermediate) On & Off the Spectrum.

You may say Simon cornering the (Book market) isn't constructive as **Practical usages** in the Market place... 'yet hey look it is a great way to advertise, meet rub shoulders then teach all that is Practical good usage theory made easy'.

Typed in **Emails** - already in format/including newly drafted.

I'd also give you in-depth details... (those Interested), simply asked of me (business Interests) customized. In mind - your designs - my ideas.

Any such Interests you wish discuss my way - makes enquiries. I am happy sending you forward plans: should Self Employment (One Day) take Root with me.

My (Electronic - **Business Cards**) so on - with in-depth details/changes... Contact info - requested.

Business Ideas all things In mention all subject too leverage, at Job centres/governments gave in Backings or non. Under analysis always. You could easily Start an

Idea your 'backed' by. Then later told it is no longer Legislation Legal. So Enthusiasm turns rhetorical. Told then, 'come'. You must be Interested in something, ((you like doing)).

Take Work/Requests, Projects you forefront me. Customized Carpentry all things made with Wood materials. Till I'm able, deciding on a Price **you feel** appropriate.

I cannot give you - **cast Iron** Guarantees in business I freely under take. I have **A.S., I think differently.**

Should you **like** my **Work** - you can spread the Word - I will log '**take Orders**' whenever I tell you I am now **Self - employed.**

Remember though wherever my path directs myself (I Work on my own). I have no partners... so speed is slow, care attention is dedication.

Should small business set a Road I follow later, take off, with flying colours. Appreciate please, a back log Orders will form an orderly Queue, or look hey you may give up your Job. Work with me.

I apologize (as to why) I am not Selling myself with the enthusiasm one seeks. ((I'd like)).

Look is only a sketch, plans I put forward, plans you hand me, job-centres (accept or don't). The climate in policy's in place can alter also. My work hard efforts, nothing is placed bedrock.

So left powerless at times - Ideas I run with.

This is not cause 'I am not Enthusiastic', I obviously am.

I try live in high Spirits, no matter my body closing down under Strain tensed.

My future plans stay healthy only kicking a penny down the road annoyed frustrated yet Smiling still. My body - my own will, only moves so far at a time. (Powers graced with or without).

Other Projects enticing small open doors at this stage, gathering slow paces at first, whilst laying bare boning foundations into my business, I have had omit. Presently from my Book. Time/space reducing your boredom.

My Business works on Principles of me Selling my Goods then I pay H.M.R.C. Once a year. Whilst keeping **close ties** with **Job Centre** - liaising with **Enterprise First.**

Pursuing Self-employment.

They'll require Working out (what Benefits) I am still, or still not Entitled too. Housing Benefit, Council Tax e.t.c.

It really is a day to day (existence), no doubt playing things by Ear (Always). You're going to run into snags problems most is likely.

Job Centre (may even decide), **I'm** better off - **going it alone...** and lifting up my decking ladders away from Job Centre moorings. Paying my own 'Housing Benefit, Rent, Council Tax' full amounts. Although risky (still remains), since Self-employment is (Risky Profit). So do I receive Benefit on those (Less Profitable Weeks & Months) making Up my short falls.

So in due time. The good plan ((Lessening a Benefit)) here, ((lessening a benefit)) there, in accordance to what's fair. In accordance to my: Weekly; Monthly; Annual Turnover Profits made. Or look simply not made.

Again lots of paperwork ((on both-sides)).

A good week in business for me is, 'I can pay my Rent'. A bad fluctuation one week one month - coming **worse**, then a system will need some - safe counter measure.

We All require Help, I only offer my hand where and when I am Authorized, Help by You.

Benefits - (taken from, or staying in 'my account'), (dependent on my earnings) In each stock month/stock year 'my small business' brings In, or simply doesn't. The way business is uncertain. Is with risk. But hey what an Adventure.

Paying Rent, so on - with 'Savings' when, business is not Good. I'd happily do we shine as, Humans. Should my Business 'not always keep head above' water, then I am lost in a **circling debate** of: (not being able) (and able too, **pay**) my **Rent. One week, One month** - Council Tax, Housing e.t.c.

My Asperger's can **cope** with a **lot** helped from a genuine source, left alone.

So using a '**Benefit system**' ((**as less** as, **I/he** can)) helping a Taxpayer or lowering the deficit. Is said helping.

Caring, (my willingness) pays in Sponsored Walks. So hey Start here.

Chapter 21.

I hear just same 'one' voice.

The way an A.S. (**hears** a **person**), he simply hears, then Sees (a message), before attempting befriend all his Others. Giving people a fair hearing, (always do), though know when caring and sharing - is not every one's game.

Heightened anxiety we assume, remember most find us rude, A.S. tied up in knots, restrains from Talking his own World, most find Odd, knowing why he must retreat back home, so I do.

The way I hear most people, is they talk with the same Monotone of voice running throughout his consecutive persons he is, rubs his consecutive others, sometimes pleasantly which is good, though still mainly to their own benefited groups.

These same Monotone of peoples that are running consecutive throughout, may be grouped into nice people, and bad people.

Not knowing their monotones or how each reacts (too you), at any given time.

Monotone people can be Lawyers, Doctors, Bankers, Secretaries, Administration staff, (P.A.s), Dentists, Retail staff, General Public, Officials - to name but a few.

Moving ((slid-en scale)) with mixed breeds, found those you're better off just walking past and Smiling or today they're approachable - blow hot and cold. Algorithms staged with unsettling Rhythms played out, with my own Smiling - Always Autistic self.

Entrepreneurial Executives wrapped up themselves thug ch-av-like behaviours blend their working monotone Executive messages inbuilt alliances, (One sound fits all people.)

N.T.s being this nice, nasty or middle road adjustments. My A.S. Unchanged gives up prediction reading situations, I Smile Happy throughout hoping acceptance is my forever Friend.

This is where, for me, problem lays in Society - you never quite know the reaction your get/give, persons on route meet. With A.S. like myself Guarantee is something we need full stop. Ways I turn Out, Always.

My Individuality is not survivable in a paper narrow World I have nothing in Common. I'd be the fool, lying to myself, just to be ((a part)) of who they want demanded, with no growth - smothered, at a very best.

To be frank with you, I'd not the motivational skills tell you ((my story)), for clearly you will denounce me, every opportunity I give, different is my Over.

I'm not about foolishly instinctively let my guard down, so undercuts me. My A.S. bridges are fragile, so protecting hard, is what I am about.

Rock crawling vermin have us at a loss, reaching for our higher ascent. Their spill/toxic words is again, not survivable cushions of air we can hang around with for to very long, we're punching for a higher intelligence, pretending unfolds around me as acceptable - is not. We just Smile, awkward agree.

The life Cycle Asperger's battles is that similar trying to distinguish extinguish the fleas around him.

Believing what 'your Others' believe, fighting their battles. Pretences you're happy with this, dispositions (where you're going, from where I belong). Those many lost Original you's. Just so making Quickened friends. And why Autistic I go it Alone, like David Banner Hulk.

The what's he, talking about people.

'**The what's - he, talking about people**', you know the ones, punching you down for everything you say wrong when following them to a T. Putting not one foot wrong. Still intimidated, under their charade - a shower of persons' indicated (look a like, people). Left shaken, left nerves. In their company.

Their Intent? - a person it leaves, strong unhappy... strong weak. At off key times, playing with selected emotions one by one. You think his your friend one moment, finding popping up disagreements. Frightened to come out your quiet zone with him... with a 100% friend club, he asks of you.

I avoid with the longest stick... as best I am able, these ego lost souls. Glorying his (same) friends, backing his 100% magnificence.

People ring-fenced in one goal, humiliating you... gives them a power keep growing taller higher, push tactic ways - shove me, push you, move over sorts. Observations, my came across, decent - descending.

Really I was seeking only a passage past you, walk past with, the least-est littlest fuzz as I humanly shall create. Friendship, on no ones terms.

Only please.

(The what's - he, talking about people), In my view - pound you, (so to be structured like them). What once was considered taboo wrong, has people catering to his folly.

I took up Guitar so too drown out a bad Spirit, left behind from (these kinds).

If you yourself (are asking the questions), **what is he, ever talking about...** smartened 'lifts in you', you get from a payment of laughter's ((you received)), you fall in line in my book totality, to persons' never making dis-aligns disassociation followings you muster friendship (an **only way In, friendship**) - built on nervous ground - (to stay), how you say... (In with you).

You are most likely over powering in your stance, as you walk towards me. Trying hard crush me like cockroach, feeling stones you carry weigh heavy - I jam my **Asperger's Ready** for **Battle Shield,** between battle fought lines. Walking away now powerless emotional no response, my wing-mirrors goodbye.

I see you again walking down a road, I use often - one day.

'Angry you', this time - was laughing and joking a walk today, with the same knuckle head others. When I said alright mate out of respect, you didn't recognize me, my baseball cap I wear. TK Maxx Sunglasses.

All I heard you say was - '**what's he talking about, who is** that **guy**'.

I carried on driving laughing smiling, turns up me Radio enjoying 2 weeks holidaying away. Lulworth Cove in Weymouth. West Country.

Moved on more. Tenting memories, Coastal Safe havens.

Untwisted away healing, Revitalizing re-plans, ((relaxing)).

You carried on smiling and laughing. With no memory no care, of pains you caused the A.S. Others.

Following in your footsteps like (child with adult), we carried on growing happy light-tunnels, places we tried sharing a respect with you. Yet Walking (with you) Alone I gave only Good Thoughts back. Our New Friendship is Good, Strong - now I am Alone.

Tension in your Area.

I get very tired when I am not allowed use my A.S. energy in my Way.

Feeling pinned down restricted in movements in an Area you live, a conformity you pretend be like them, yet in many regards, is why you became the loner. Taking only a Scenic Path, me accepting smiling, (then you angry we smiled), is a world in which (you ask to see change), yet heavily pinned down in this change leaves us again awkward non changed.

For we know ((this change)), any change... only benefits those who have already dominated an area, in every step walked. No matter of pretty pictures we are told - ((sits present)), working for the good.

Many don't realize (Change seekers), will remain at odds, with Non Changing man. Change seeking people instantly are, associated, as the Hard Workers.

Non Changing man Works Hard - his only difference; is, he Won't Change. He likes who he is. Nevertheless by osmosis, it is considered cause his Non Changing, his also Non Hard Working. A label tags. Like Insects, lay eggs.

My Reasoning's strictly conform as: (non Changer - Hard-worker, frozen in time, of Spectrum disorders)… looked at Oddly.

A mind philosophy my A.S. Is, can't simply stem the flow (for the convenience of), your ever grows - controlling Communities. Wanting things for you in their community you share not one same love for. Put simply (It is not you).

Made feel abandoned if you don't fit, we stop doing Well - trashed again.

Smiling along pretending every things OK - yet decreeing odd. New make shift policies 'we are said to - **look like**' - is not (me).

A.S. Sees, very little elbow room for Error, to be an Open easy going Human being.

I noticed how passionate our governance are, working in Communities, 'big-hand shake'. Yet for all CCTV Cameras, technologies available, you hardly ever see them used, to the fullest.

Sure Speed Cameras on our much loved Motorways, they crop up more than Daisies field. Taxes Revenues 'they pull-in'. Topping up Gov spend pots, contributes.

The whole thing to me is - nothing short - one big fat

soggy Ice Cream Cornet, slung out high Executives Car window. Unsightly Curb pavement - Melts away, while high end management Executives man, is our look up too role model. 'We all must shape'.

It is not our Governments faults we still feel inadequate in our so called Community's to them who strut around. Owning every last inch of territory, ((that to share))... in the Community, and strut the same, only has you looking like the - ((One look)) - tailored for: 'One all only Uniforms'.

Life in an Ideal World.

Life in an Ideal World is the continual Happiness you keep 'keep on become strong, in your Happiness', when all 'different and sames people', pull their Weight, not to dishearten you or another other.

Moreover - ((we have seen enough)).

Start turning on those Happy Switches, would yea please.

Let people 'give people', as much time sensitivity, 'turning around one neat circle, their life's around', so yes you hear the other Shoe drop, walking in-line your rhythmic other foot.

So pleased, - kept good Rhythm steady beat is hardly fought with, holding him our A.S. me back. Normal back, who suffer same situations as A.S.

Whilst his brought in-line real deal Care; he shows you for your patience A.S. come N.T.

Decontamination. This really is the end. Thank-you my Readers.

So here, my Boat comes in rested moored. I thank you my Readers In support of my Books.

Just Reading a little bit each Night, on a Tea-break, is took same brave walks Asperger people, show lost in constantly.

You surely can hide with a Loving World - in the best scenario, though still feel an Isolation a Loneliness, only you have Power.

With A.S. you make a great deal of breakthrough s, though always all battles have us where we made the Starts.

Listen to us today - forgotten easily next week.

It is ((not British Values)) - I look for as A.S.

((It is, Asperger Values)).

The saddest part for myself taken on writing my book of this magnitude, is knowing when I walk away from all I say, passing a fellow passer by on his travels, he'll still forever know me as only the Stranger.

Thank you for journeying my personal World within Asperger's catered - let us treat all fashioned A.S. N.T.s like great Authors, you tried explaining they were.

Most of all - love the Author you turn into.

So you are Unique. Special.

So you are different. So you are openly you.

This book was written from my heart, emended grit determination.

I have been Simon with A.S. Amplified. Spectrum. A.S.

Alternate. Strategic. A.S.

Always. Simon. A.S.

Asperger's is like: ((The Indian Space Race)), finally dreams we don't struggle in as hard is our tried plan since certain advances empower our backing, confidence rest you.

An Asperger's dream is not won through preaching, 'won by choice' by general ordinary people who think in terms reasoned fair. And nothing but nothing more to add before walking with education that is us - allowed to be us. My Individual Way I share presented.

Never seen, an endings - satisfied. New debates lead incur new debates, completing all covered ground is virtually impossible so remains good opener; to further your talks, later books planned.

I heard a great teacher once say to me, the Simplest fundamental Principles, 'are more often the hardest' - when take on-board digest you do; since you've really got to ((slow down, in ways)) you're not use to connecting. So back in fundamental land hurting your mind till speed is gained.

There comes a point in an Unfinished Life a book must end - so I decided to put my stop in here.

My fountain pen words 'is where I live', laid with battle shields laid down - piled up neatly not required no more.

I wrote within love pain awkward of canter.

Similar in me diagnosed under this title; is your Conclusion.

I Rested you an A.S. Soul I am.

Asperger's refers my law I am principled In.

Asperger's I further you my Education furthering your reading.

Asperger's is fun & healthy.

Asperger's is Simon.

Acknowledgements.

I would like to **thank:**

My Mum:

My Mum. Always there for all us children, me eldest of 4. My 2 brothers, Sister, my step dad Paul, my mum's stepson - and grandchildren. She's a good friend to all family - friends.

My Mum along with my step dad Paul show good advocates to all people, smiling through the quiet pain. Pain seen in them, pain seen others, yet smiling help others - pain hurts no more. Absorb soaked up - spread thins out, (carry) - what pain is left, seal tight in cotton silk cloth, tied in on all 4 corners. Happiness love Family's strength. Indian chief strong.

My Mum's wealth - not sat in bank earning Interest, unspent without second thoughts what gains they may crank up. Instead unfolded relaxed cloth - Mum, Paul alike. Take me out Meals. Phone check I'm OK. 1st one's there, situations with solutions, awkward asking persons' in other Norms I'd not do so.

Some people can't show outbound happy Joy - for they feel they must - (stay our Grey picture) or people won't like them ((when they're happy)). Only when they harness Over open Grey are they loved.

My Mum is tower of strength within an otherwise sensitive soft gentle body shell. She wins through us all, Joseph's amazing Technicolor dream-coat wise.

All human Spiritual beings - come about of ageless, uniformed universal in today's togetherness with hindsight - as one likeness - yet your mum humanities gold's future, your plans. Someone different you alone See.

The magic my childhood was: we lived ((forever)) and ever.

Ageless life within this World remains, I stay misunderstood. Unfinished for my truth won only my best friends whom Struggled, unrewarded, sneered at scoffed an ignorance matters not. We got each Other.

More than this a loving Mum. Just plainly forgiving not rewarded Smiles joy.

My Mum best - explained me - ((best once)) - saying she know how find real Simon - missing return scents, drawing Home. We simply - mess up his room.

Then he knows where everything is.

My Mum happily is your Nobody for you, until Someone happily knows, she's more than Somebody. Whilst Caring enough becomes lesser, giving you higher Praise, my mum's forward plan with You.

Loves quiet wisdom is my Mum. XX Paul Murley. XX

I would like to **thank:**

My Dad.

Who has always been there for me in life. Not always airing/sharing thoughts, though Happy. My dad puts ((care love first)), accepts found differences, shapes of same - with generally found easy going free shrugs Forever green Forests.

Keeping a kept happiness (for others) - runs in front of himself. Longs as others - ((are OK)) - then my dad's taking shorter straw. No grumbling no fuss.

Asking not more of others than they physically can perform. Just go at your pace is all I've known.

Mannerisms, professionalism is my Dad. Completing Jobs, without half moon's Intelligent eyes peering over Glasses required. Wearing only half moon specs good deeds requires.

No Fame required, no designer labels required, just wears smarter clothes. His World looks, smells great.

No matter what stage - high success, barely making it my Dad kept an equal love running through all my joys.

Days out fishing, flask of coffee and sandwiches. Sandy step mum, made my dads' wife - or odd games of Snooker here and there.

My Dad has been with me forever - is always saying, here you go Son here's a Tenner or here's a Fiver, or like you know - here's twenty squid.

It may not be much my Dad ((say)), but it's all I got. Easter eggs at Easter, never forgotten or rarely.

Best of all my Dad and my Mum (Eileen) gave me an Identity to Christmas what it should be like - then look like Christmas Is as a young child my Special gift I remember. Excited feelings in my Stomach helps my love as developed adult I am.

Calm happier Times - Christmas when was, your World you remembered, excitement I once built, was an energy you find hard to say. (Yes this is how described), places in time when life was good - hard to re-in-act, this energy in those bringing forwards comes only Once.

The Spirit magic of Christmas, Special people.

Helps calmness, love of attitude, my Child Christmas Spirit in you, ((over come)) - better then I'd guess, had they not shown a love at all over coming - is why Christmas is Gold Red Green's God's Special Christmas Colours.

I thank you my Dad and Mum (Eileen) for what I believe best only definition of Gifted love. A teaching not taught - but given - reacted genuine sincerity gave love.

Thank you Dad I remember Special Moments.

Dad/Sandy - Newell. XX

I wish also Sandy step mum my Dad's wife a (fast recovery) she broke her neck tripping on a handbag strap from all accounts. And am sure she'll be back to her good fighting self in no time. Mobilising back her old self, Little house on the prairie. The Walton's. Bonanza. Country music. Healing soon. Your a good person. God speed Simon. XX

I would like to **thank:**

My Uncle Uncle Bert. Aunty Aunty Aud.

Thanking you Uncle uncle Bert and Aunty Aud.

Strength your presence dominates my soft love felt - no physical presence, walks in us better.

Thought of in moments quiet - loved normal decent people, by all who share far away from Valleys Wales and those close to hand.

Uncle Bert, it goes without saying, you're our guiding Star Bethlehem with Aunt Aud.

You bring conscience to a Family, who move in beloved Wisdoms we call upon.

Made look simple remedies - makes all the Family follow your lead, and they do smile a little Joy.

When life proves too Political on Average people there are better Ways. Happy am I under slow casual progress. Kindness Uncle Bert, Aunt Aud emulates gladly through my Years is me in boat behind following foot steps. Humble, Noble then fair.

Uncle Bert you're very Caring Soulful Man. Giving Man.

Once opening Granddad Arthur's fridge door a few moons ago, back in Leopold St. I see newspaper lined wooden trays, cork - Rag Worms - Granddad kept cool for Fishing

- in with the Milk and Cheese.

It made me shudder yet at the same time it felt right. Felt senses, smells - Granddad's house.

Uncle Bert from buying us toys when we younger. Uncle Bert - Mouse Trap by M.B. Games.

To Action Man. ((In old traditional Diving gear - lead Boots - and those old rounded coppery brass, bronze heavy helmet masks, deep sea divers wore traditionally back in later days)).

To Christmas/Birthday Cards, money sent more than generously, not just to me, the wider family too.

You have more than done your bit for this Family Uncle Bert. Makes us grateful - better when we can be seen helping you out, just with the odd email here and there, ((Letters)). Visiting you - the feeling of Wales, Welsh flag.

Uncle Bert good old days. Clear blue open World. It once was stood lost in time still - Universal Rhythm.

A feeling one could breathe. Open door World. Lost in time, many many moons - hard to re-live, recreate re-enact a time special. A 1,000 piece jigsaw is only built once - special worlds gone.

Car Journey's blue skies - those days lasting forever.

Days - weeks - months - years rolled as (One day) - sounds of - ((((Forever)))).

Time gone.

Happy I am - in my own peace and quiet - hearing only passing odd Aeroplane - the blue, blue Skies on Sunny days. Yachts in our traditional past - history disconnected from Grey World History is our History, separate History logged as written my cares.

Forever open fields the people we forgot we were. The days we once could show openly, strongly.

Readers Digest books, manuals I read, from my Dad's

collection.

Workbenches handed down my Dad, I made many a Carpentry projects upon: pipe racks, magazine racks - you name it.

Kevin surprised me - downloaded a Black and White Photo via Email, I keep in my living room of Granddad at his Workshop preparing a ((Car spray)). The purpose of your journey down here Portsmouth - 7 day stay - back in the '60s.

Kevin uploaded also a recent photograph of you and Aunty Aud - I'll simply frame soon.

God/bless, thank you. Love from Simon XX

I would like to **thank:**

Kevin Kearn, and his wife **Win.**
My Uncle Bert's friend my friend. Kevin is my Uncle Bert's friend from the Wirral.

It is very rare in life I find connection with another. Kevin has a power, a gift - set record straight in no uncertain terms - making burnt toast feel like it's bread & butter soldiers dipped with runny egg soldiers.

Kevin's words of a word-smith, folds, polishes, hardens, cleans, strengths - like sword, 1,000 times. And why I made my conscious choice - asked kindly may I enter my Written Letter received now my Testimonial - at front of this book 2.

Aspiring Influences me, view points cherished.

Words like: 'poverty of Spirit' for instance - Kevin helped me see.

Kevin gave me good reference to my First book, testimonial, even with my novice Author approach as I came, bad Grammar, uncomfortable Autistic feelings.
I left some Readers Well Read. Kevin looked beyond this, my first Take, waiting first Struggles were part my Chasten with you here Today, belief Struggles

Intermediate raised my upped Author.

Thank you Kevin - thank you.

I have never met Kevin though Kevin explains:

Having spoken of you Simon with your Uncle Bert and Aunt Aud so often - it feels as if we know each other already, Kevin wrote in a lovely letter to me.

Kevin has known my Uncle Bert/Aunt Aud - over Sixty years, so he gets over, sees them whenever the opportunity arises.

In beautifully crafted letter to me a while back, Kevin explains he came to Portsmouth Leopold Street, off from Albert Rd of Southsea in early 1960s. He must have been 19. He stayed a week with my Granddad, Resident in Leopold Street. The sole purpose of journey was to Spray up my Uncle Bert's Car, from my understanding.

Uncle Bert's brother my Granddad, had a car Mechanics small Business - and Kevin stayed at my Grandmother's house in Leopold Street.

This made me chuckle. Kevin goes on to explain he had very vivid memories of that wonderful week, he spent with my Grand father, Arthur Newell.

Though one memory that won't leave Kevin was my Granddad at his Workshop, then going on break with him for what he, my Granddad, described as a 'board meeting' somewhere. When Kevin got to this meeting 'the board' was in fact headed down the Pub - the pub's dartboard meeting!

You understand the funny side, I tell you my Granddad an Alcoholic.

Back in them days 'Alcoholics' were, dare I say, traditionally normal - the real fisherman's spirit my Granddad was. A World when men were men.

Old traditional names - in feelings of like - Lenny. Ron. George. Reg were sort of names you might picture my Granddad's - cronies - friends envisaged.

Rough neck good Naval types - Trawler fisherman strong personalities. Worked, graphed fingers, 'real people'.

Kevin showed me an old picture back in Time with my Granddad and the guys who Worked with him - Naval bloke types from my seen and heard understanding, ((my Dad, Bob Newell)) informed me.

So On-line black and white Photo Kevin was kind enough forward on.

Photo I treasure.

Captured spirit not retrievable in the timelessness. Priceless, having my Granddad back with Us.

A love lost memories, only Granddad made a place energize soft flickers glowing light. Green glass Tilley lamp his Character, just one element expressing.

The Photo is of Granddad with the guys at his Workshop (ready to spray Uncle Bert's car). My Dad says young person situated in black & white - to your back right - might be him possibly.

I want thank you Kevin one last time testimonial at front book means a lot. Shall stay with me always,

Forever. God bless, thank-you Kevin. X

Helen, Kevin's daughter of Hoylake:

From little girl, Helen adopt Aunty Aud/Uncle Bert's (care love).

Still to this day.

I not met Helen myself - however I forwarded her copy of my 1st book The Plain Truth, is my only met connection. Thank-you Helen. Simon. x

I would like to **thank:**

My Step Dad, Paul John Murley.

My step dad is simple man hiding complex intelligence

he easily could shown World's arena - the many personalities we converse to meet. Paul doesn't require to stand tall. He doesn't require the discerning chats that make men - feel Important.

Paul copes with wisdoms he articulates, by turning all mathematics of life - on their upside downs - on their heads.

Sure Paul can go off In a huff, though after a walk gone few hours - watching the calm tide Paul comes home energized.

Paul has much he himself copes with, in the built free humans we live out. His leg has not been said normal since an accident going back moons ago, hence limping walks. Non complaining for the best part.

We are human though, and so Paul fights through - when all situations become a complete gut-full.

Paul thinks with his heart. He loves most people equally - his best love is for the family.

Nothing is too much for Paul. You need a lift - you got it.

You want help Moving home - you got it. You just wish someone dress up with you go to Restaurants, Weatherspoons, not a problem.

You want a day out fishing - hey meet you at 6am.

I have lots of Shopping I can't manage, on me self. You got it again, Paul helps.

Paul no matter of the pains illnesses we all break under - he'll take you the time. He never gives up, cause a new strength, climbs on in on board support.

Paul is a young-man, in an older body.

I can see the pains pushing through him, when he himself - just has had a level up - 'to here' - gut full.

People love Paul more than physical expressions leaves their clues.

The best ((gift)) in essence, is he lives in happy.

Paul has this amazing belief system. He believes in people - and without speaking it. He has, how you say, this sort of holy spirit guidance, not surprised when others are reaching the high goals he casually takes it back in his stride. Almost a cocky, cockney nice of see, 'I told you so'.

He loves people at the end of the day. In the before and after Successes. His presence didn't wither many reach struggles - and rose.

Thank - you Paul. Simon. XX

I would like to **thank:**

My God Mother.

Aunty Bet - Betty Rosser, aged 84 - 87 or so, with as much fight in her still (to this day) as in her younger years.

Aunty Bet in my book - ((has never grown old)), it's only structured years saying they past gave her recorded age. Spirit she is glad - never ages.

My God Mother is my rare - one in every Billion people you meet on this short stay on Earth that is all American Humanistic down to her very very loved by others - core. Soulful, playful, strong, happily loud - smoothing company.

Aunty Bet reminds me Soul of this Family, like my Uncle Greg, Caring live by her up lifting presence, American in Britain 'Character' that makes Aunty Bet - Aunty Bet.

She's our Aunty Bet.

My greatest past memories remembers Aunty Bet was 'Partys' Family member Aunty Bet held from, young life forever child ((party & games)), a good World - perfect trance I was.

Games like (Simple Simon) - where you had follow correct

Colour sequences in orders they flashed - you then repeated.

Other games we played at party's ranged anything from like:

Ker Plunk ((marbles & straws)).

Major Morgan electronic game.

Speak & Spell.

Pin the tail on the Donkey. Blind man's buff.

Musical Chairs. Pass the Parcel - name a selected few.

Remembering flash backs, sweet spot memories I leak.

Running up and down (on Aunty Bet's Landings) - 'winding Stairs' from top to bottom - middle to top - back down and up. Towers of flights & flights of stairs.

Each ((Landing)) - takes you to other flats, on same each Landing, building with varying mysterious levels - Nightingale Road of Southsea Portsmouth.

Nightingale Road's Carpet patterns were traditional pearl-tailed like yin yang swirl shapes en trenched. Blues all shades -purples - turquoises, of a '70s era long ago, designs of '70s Colour. Aunty Bet's high, many Storey Flats - atmospheric feelings, large mirrors furniture feel good - white leather suites unobtainable recreates.

As child I played marble games on patterned Carpet that never stopped fascinating or jumped from one pattern to the next. I was safe on certain parts of the carpet, childhood imagination - maybe an A.S. child, early signs.

Party ((Spreads)) Aunty Bet laid on for people through the years, is one extra such memory you can't replace. The energy of the '70s & '80s - was my real open breathing World - leave your back door open, it's a real Summer's day.

This energy is something you search the rest of your

placement on earth for. Oxygen in Lungs spirit hazed comes only once in life, the good memories, mercury rested in thermometer, past time magic of childhood, cloud formations long past, re-live a place homes escape when really down, I feeling low.

Our Uncle Paul and Roger Rosser - Aunty Bets Son's from America - always bought us ((Presents back)) - from U.S.A. whenever they were over visiting United Kingdom. ((Baseball Glove)) Pyjamas Bunny suits.

My ((Baseball Glove)) - had that all American smell in the leather - I treasured that Glove. It went missing without me realizing, aware only now broken it gone. Years later. More importantly losing my ((One Glove)) isn't lost.

Catching still my one heart's Glove.

Aunty Bet said best is - Robin William' strength, that when we ((got Home)) - from family visits 'her living energy' stayed with us forever.

Smells in my clothes. Attach.

You leave persons days on days later, only fragrances you associated activities remains long gone - 'lives.'

Development ways we grew up - turned out people we became. Reasons part and parcel who you this day - and moving. I Remains today weaker signals, with no way back, protective dusts who you'll Stay.

Yesterday's World gone. Thank you Aunty Bet. XX

I would like to **thank:**

My Sister Hayley.
New Born baby, **Sebastian.** Antony. Shaun. Kerridge.

Hayley always been there for me through out my life. She's always there for anyone seems everyone.

Very generous by Nature, she projects goes beyond calls

of duty in all she does (Presents she buys) - persons' through Years, both Birthdays Christmases certain Specialized Occasions.

I Wrote a Song back a while - called ((Hayley)) to thank Hayley for her hard work.

I have intentions 'release' on Music Acoustic Session C.D. by Simon, along with many Songs I Wrote for Acoustic Guitar - Hayley's Song Inclusive.

All Songs I wrote/write - extends my people under Spectrum's Rainbow, a backbone running dedication my first ever book The Plain Truth.

Hayley Inspirations with others myself, kind in her Stride Sister. And how you might expect your Sister image to be had you - had one yourself. Perfect Hologram Imagination brought elements together, then your collective Sister Want-age Symmetrical Butterfly is Hayley.

She will laugh along with you in her giggling bubbling at ease Nature, she helps others over the expenses of seeing fulfilment pocketed for One, yet gave with Soul to One. Many across unique we wish grow different bonus with togetherness you wink horizon water pebbles, skimmed on beache's Tide.

This type of messaging: 'if all people were same' then in this instance - yes would be a better place uniquely different.

Hayley's moved on in life.

So must we all.

Thank you. Love Hayley and Sebastian.

Brother Simon. XX

I would like to **thank:**

My Daughter: **Natasha Chloe Patrisha Lee.**

Natasha was Reunited with me - three years ago.

Great see her under my own terms my eyes, 16 years life both miss out - time lost.

Natasha is an Artist - likes to Draw/Paint.

Her talent surpasses her calm collective mannerisms.

Natasha's talent amount efforts she pours within her Drawings, effortless not a problem, walking Strife of Greatness - soaks up energies took set times in place.

Apart of the World, or her latest in friends, she is not rewarded so much way Easy going natures carry us. How University Lecturer's persons' of Importance, protect lights in gifts, constant looking after, if to grow to strengths, height. Ambition drive saturated deserving.

Congratulated traced back flows, freelance Artists Natasha works In. Lost Originators go unrecognized, lost with reborn, new mixed my best Artists, friendly very giving never no problem Artist with Influence Inspired.

Note good Readers:

Artwork on request **by Natasha Lee.**

Natasha's Pictures - Art Paintings for **SALE:**

Paintings - Drawn Pictures - Artwork - Portraits - on Requests.

Hinting what she'll tackle is not my Decision. I am sure versatile adaptive most Requests, though I cannot speak for her here: Little/much Work - availability - is in her Time Timings moods of Today tomorrow. Saying Yes, saying No Artists freedom establish I leave Open.

Pick from already - on Sale Paintings.

Natasha's Drawings from I gather, Art Work is On Sale now.

((On Request Ideas Pictures)) - you'd like share with her. Ideas set scene Living-room, Bedroom, Bathroom, Hallway come as may.

You may contact me via my Email address: smn_nwll@Yahoo.co.uk

I Pass-on Requests.

Contact Tasha direct on her face-book page typing:

Tasha's Art for **Sale.** Her prices you'd discuss with her.

As the Artist Tasha may freely turn down requests, she may be delighted of the Work. I am not to know this, where Time Stages of Life shroud Today's new makeup.

She may jot your name down, for later in the day appointments, she may say I stopped Selling, put Stop to Requests, sorry. She may show Thundering Keen. She may decide freely Always.

Thank you for your understanding.

My way of helping.

Take Special care Natasha - Good luck Simon, Dad XX

I would like to **thank:**

My **2 Brothers: Matthew/Michael.**

Their 2 Partners, **Jaime Newell/Katy Robinson** includes their Children.

2 Brothers grown up Men now, not just loved by me, they're loved by those new Families they chose, from early ages - with today's, saying yes here's my Only Ones I want to stay join creation Old/New Family. Families split, stay, moved on, love Stays. Happy Days.

Michael and Matthew are (Close brothers), I'm Big outer brother recoiled my way Grace.

Perhaps that's why Love Works, cause it has no rules - we just accept wheat blows through hands of Christ.

Both Michael and Matthew, I think fair say, Love their Football. Food. They put /shoulder - a lot into Life.

Matthew Is contract Worker 'Electrician' is away out Falkland Islands a lot - 3 Months here - 4 Months there. As when Work becomes available Matthew goes. Matthews Talks with me enthusiasms Meaningful XX

Michael Works as a Postman. Always High Spirited. His Laughter Inner Humour Archangel carries Good.

Good Dad with his Children. XX

Jaime Newell: Loyalism Addresses people with correct Tones. x

Katy Robinson: Bounds Welcome certitude exuberant insightful. x

I would like to **thank:**

My Nanny Newell ((Betty)).

I was close Nanny Newell, especially from age 12 to 14 - up to late teen years.

I made a habit to see my Nan regular as clockwork, I used the excuse to clean my Nan's brass, bronze, but Secretly I loved our talks.

My Nan had Arthritis crippling her hands, made movements - from into the Sofa Chair and Out - very awkward uncomfortable, you see my Nan's pain. We would wait with her till present pain passed, especially in just slightest moves, everything was cramped painful. Although I couldn't feel Nan's pain, I could see it.

I only know twentieth of what my Nan went through in physical her body, all whiles bravely smiling through seen pain, she was enshrouded of - whilst others were helpless to do much, just sink our heads hands in clasped lap sympathize.

Most my deepest remembrances kept thoughts - my Nan close - was tracing back times she lived at Keswick Avenue. Copnor Portsmouth - with Uncle Biff who was retired Marine, Ex Serviceman my Nan took In. He soon from all accounts as I understand it, was known set forward as our Uncle Biff ever since.

Shouting out his favourite line - ((Shut that blo**y door)) pushing it shut with his walking stick.

Uncle Biff was loved by many.

Hard terms just say Uncle Biff was regimented - he was but really this man was the backbone of the family 'Love the likes' - I'll never - be able to explain this beautiful power.

My Uncle Biff's bedroom was fill chock-a-block Air Fix Models, and that's no warping exaggeration ((he loved making Crafts)) - painting up Airplanes. Fire Engines. Boats. Tanks. He was an enthusiast you could say - blimey. Wow.

The pipe smells of Uncle Biff regimented as part his character.

My Uncle Biff loved anything to do with History. I know this the way he glared

over 50 mins a book on History I took to my Nan's place once. The History was of 'Bodiam Castle' - moated in 14th Century East Sussex - my Dad took us out on a day trip there just few days before.

Nan lived also with my Aunty Jenny and Uncle Greg, her daughter my Aunty. Hilsea Gatcombe Park. Portsmouth. Later In life.

Nan with her hands failing still found courage to Knit best-est of the best - Knitted Jumpers.

My Nan made ((Jumpers for all our Family)) - on a knitting machine upstairs in Gatcombe Park where she lived - top and bottom rooms of back extension.

My Dad's side of the Family my Nan had Polish Jewish blood lines assent and so you see my Nan in likeness - the Plum Homemade Jams Nanny made, the Cod liver Oils Home from Home.

Nan had this favourite Rhyme Rhythm she always Sang to us Children was:

I'm going to have **those belly** on the **Spots. B**elly on the Spots. Belly on the Spots. So it repeated.

The air opened around my Nan people could breathe in my Nan's Home from Home love. She played Organ long ago - and was not such a bad Musician herself I learn.

Walking into Keswick Ave Copnor - I fondly remember an Organ to my left, Cactus plants, stairs ahead Living-room, right - dining room leads kitchen left.

My Nan whenever you had a problem she sorted it out for you, from lending people money, to Saving money for me in a Jar - like my personal accountant.

To giving good sound advice. Home truths. This resonated through bubble clear strength - we made sure her message was understood.

My Nan was awesome good Cook, not surprising with my Granddad once on board in her life before she divorced past moons.

Nan loved growing Homemade Strawberries white pots garden positioned - out in back garden. The Fishes pond broken path slabs pave cobbled effective angles. Vehicle Tire halves made black Flowerpots.

Gnomes were flaking under bad weather, so I said, Nan I would clean up wire brush, and Oil paints.

2 weeks later I surprise nanny with the good works. I couldn't wait, excited to show her. Though I came across reserved contains hidden real Excitement.

My Nan had a Weather Vane Man wind direction pointer Garden creak swing chair spiritual good Character - broken pathways, worked Nan's garden.

Brandy, Nan's Uncle Biff's Bulldog, early lost rolling days love clean.

I will - still do - miss my Nan.

Hopes with Aunty Paddy. Happy out pain in Delight.

Love Stay Nan Newell. Simon XX

I would like to **thank:**

My Step brother: Anthony Murley Deacon/Priest.
Currently in Birmingham. Doing us - admiration.

Anthony is what an Englishman Portraits with cherry on cake, nibbling around the pastry, before divulging the complete cake.

Anthony plays his part as my Step brother very well to a T. His Love is sentiments meant listens merciful, happily happy to be just Anthony. No more.

People take to Anthony for good reason - he is sourced from genuine.

Hayley my sister brother's closely, chemistry way you might want your normal World Sing-out, let's connect. Present giving so fourth.

Anthony Works hard though you'd hardly appreciate so, an Outer easy going Charm.

Thank-you Anthony. Prayers God's Good. Amen. Simon X

I would like to **thank:**

My Granddad Arthur Newell.
Gone fishing Other side Green Turquoises missed Stay shadows.

Thank you taking me Fishing Granddad as a young boy over 35 years ago. It's funny isn't it Granddad, cast minds back as far plated priceless traditional memories housed.

Your glow humanistic I search for Granddad, finding this match I've failed, it's not something you can replica Granddad. You to me were man's model, real Rolex watch.

Something rubbed off in 'you' to me, between the Special Moments we shortly shared. And why? I fight my corners under your guidance from the rocks clashing - heavens pointing - ladle within my heart follow you these days, with added A.S.

I'm happy this way around.

In basic form traditional freedoms, is not a taught class in Schools, Colleges or Universities. That grows beloved then teaches 'all at the same time', this approach has only one Root, something taught, felt, lived out (you to me) Granddad were.

For all your faults/problems, I found it very easy to say this is what an intelligent man will look like.

A fisherman of tradition.

Your methods, your home-made remedies approaches you worked with. Home-made lures, rigs and knots. Making your own lead weights, cast moulds you engineered. Experienced 'welder' in handiness of projects - saving money.

Prove not all things bought expensive had straight seals of approval you mustered over-hard Granddad. Real Hobbies, techniques stronger durable than of fisherman with all the (fancy degrees), all the Gear. Proof enough old and traditional wins hands down.

What is more, direct from sources the heart energies better work patterns. More on point just being nothing more than what a Granddad is said to feel like - you were plainly you.

I shall always remember my Granddad - associated smells objects. Apple tree at bottom of garden, this tree the hallmarks feel of old Leopold Street. Shed to my left, old style shack outside toilet under shed's canopy - Armitage Shanks - heavy toilet chain.

Shed windows made from ((bubble wrap)) 'I loved popping the bubbles.' Old arch ((back in time tools)), too rusted to use. Saws hanging up ready for refurbishment cleans reconditioned in your time you set out.

Freedom that was freedom - back in them days... of live forever much time on your hands, the black cat bendy tail dominating the garden in her home, tail jammed in door - hence bendy tail. Rocking Chair.

The 1977 Silver Jubilee Street Party's, green tiled pubs stain glass misty cloudy logo pub windows, people smoking in bars, a pint in one hand - half inch froth heads, paper beer mats, Spirits of long gone - back in time.

Granddad was comfortable in clothes you wore traditional caramel, browns, green colours - brown buttons big size.

Shoes, safety pins - braces holding up trousers, meant look poor on outsides company others yet inside, when asked dress-up to Nines, you smelt like A-real man Granddad, tough rugged look, clean trousers, attractively shabby lint off Suit, brushed up tidy, pressed shirt. You asked next door neighbour Iron mayn't surprise, whilst you were busy say making fishing traces ready boat-fish Granddad.

Cuff links, buffed shoes, old spice, trilby hat.

You were so graceful, relaxed intelligence 'you had'. We know when a man like you granddad strong, good fishing hands, climb high Crow's Nest my heart family others.

A firm handshake grip that meant something. Forever missed.

Marvellous handmade Wedding cakes.

Crabs walking, boat fresh caught Kitchen everywhere.

Kitchen sink - side boards.

Few memories my mum remembers you by, I heard her say.

Silly things - smells, sounds, Brut aftershave, soap on a rope, old style bath tubs Victorian, 1p Back Returned used Bottle Caps Saved.

Granddad remembers.

When a Granddad Great in the oils - character comes along, 'it's a once in a Blue moon experience' - you are my Granddad.

I loved you great expressively. Simon XX

I would like to **thank:**

Nassar Kessell (Lib Dem) friend of mine Sister Hayley.
Nassar one of few good people left in this world - unique specimen - proper regular person, that is not just a run of Mill.

Nassar reminds me an old fashioned Car where you pull the Choke out - damn, Choke's broken 'so what do you do?' Yes, right - you stick a couple Clothes Pegs on - hold position retracting, the car's Choke. Hold Character Nassar's Look.

I Met Lord Mayor of Portsmouth she was Ms Lynne Stagg sat by Nassar, Guildhall Square - Meeting he Introduced me relaxed ease talking with Lynn Nassar.

Posed a question - when he said, is your Second book grand Date?

Thank-you Nassar. Time, Help Took grateful.

Good Ways deserves spot in Dictionary made of you.

Thank you so much Nassar. Simon X

I would like to **thank:**

My Nan and **Grandad Kelly.((Bill** and **Hilda)).**
Nan and Grandad on my mum's side. My Dad's side left Earth higher Places.

So that's ((four people)) - isn't it?

You think as younger person, your Nan and Grandad will be there always, like we remain Sheltered forever Status. Sadly we all reach Time move through Nicer Doors, completed our missions Earth's playground. We are dismissed, relieved duty move on regardless of good fortresses awaiting your New Company.

Jesus, when he paid for all our Sins on Cross, forgave Zealots such as Barabbas.

Jesus paid ultimate price. I, Simon bend on knees ask might he forgive, I seen error my Ways, start a New. You see none come close - our true King Jesus.

Thank you ((Jesus Christ)) - looking after my 2 Nan - 2 Grandads.

Amen. Shalom.

Grandad Kelly loved his Cricket and Golf.

Together, on ((Barton's Green field)), Wakeford's Way Havant - upon visits we played.

Grandad loved push bikes - cycled everywhere - even to the Pub - The Fox. ((No longer there is a One Stop store presently)).

Nanny Kelly was always Knitting. She loved her Snooker, no one Interrupted when the Snooker was On, especially if Steve Davis was playing, or Dennis

Taylor.

Nanny Kelly traditionally loved Tea, and so still used Tea Leaves with a Tea Strainer.

Grandad Kelly, something I look back I see my Grandad's brown/grey trousers - wearing Reflective Cycling Trouser Clips.

My Grandad Kelly was gentle Happiest Soul.

He always see the good in everything.

Loved to Read. Very Intelligent wise-man you'd hardly know Jolly Company Family regarded.

Love with you Nan/Grandad Kelly. Amen XX

I would like to **thank:**

All my Uncles and Aunties.

Aunty Jenny Uncle Greg Dowse. Aunty Jenny supportive computer posts, general speaks Well welcome relax.

Stay Over weekends visit my Younger self Jenny Greg I stay, Kensington Rd. Swap Stamps with Cousins Nick & Michelle look forwards.

Uncle Greg head of regards concern family. Sandals - New Forest - Family estate Car - Warmth. XX

Aunty Beverley and Uncle Peter Burgess.

Aunty Kim and Uncle Ian Newell.

Aunty Pat and Michael Ryan.

Aunty Kath Hooley.

Aunty Linda and Uncle Mick Kelleher.

Uncle Des. Great Golf man. X

I would like to **thank:** All my Cousins.

Nicholas Dowse. (Harmsworth.) X

Michelle Dowse.

The brilliant **Hannah Rocks.** (Cousin.) X

The Sincere **Joanne Buchanan** (Cousin.)

Russell Buchanan X

I would like to **thank:**

Pay Special Gratification too **Adam Windebank - James Windebank. X**

Gary Newell (Cousin) and Girlfriend **Sarah Cooper. X**

I would like to **thank:**

Connor Cooper. X

Kerry and **Jack Newell** (Cousins.) **X**

I would like to **thank:**

(Cousins.) **X**

Shaun and Maria Kelleher.

Chris and Rob Kelleher (Nicki Kelleher.)

Michelle and Paul Hooley.

Kevin and Tony Kelleher.

I would like to **thank:**

Eve Mountifield and Vernon. X

Friends/family. Mark - Amber Broomhead.

Eve takes time likes posts - on my computer, thank you's I say here: granted Today's allowance Thank you.

I would like to **thank:**

Kirsty and Matt Bartlett. Friends X

Sharps Copse - junior school; my good friends on computer.

I would like to **thank:**

Melinda Coffelt Social media friend from Jacksboro Texas America.

Melinda always helps me with nice things. She says - comments I grow with - walking better friends - Sky placed. Simon X

I would like to **thank:**

Roger Vincent Palmer: of Copnor Portsmouth.

Who passed on from this World. 2004. Summer time.

Roger and I would love having a beer, playing darts, in the kitchen 501. Around the board.

We enjoyed Fishing trips (fishing the Tide-up), camping Van, taking the Canoe out along Eastney to South Parade Pier. In Portsmouth Hampshire. Games down Snooker club fun. Miss you Roger dodger.

Thank you for fun we had Roger. Simon X

I would like to **thank:**

John Thompson and Irish Mick (Michael). My 2 Best-est friends at Mill House Hostel at the time.

I would like to **thank:**

Jennifer Smith. My Sister's friend, mine. Generous by default outward bound Star. x

Mikala 'Spudy' Aquilina Batatinha.

My Sister's friend, mine. Lively in goods adjusting, helpful, hard working, open /private. x

I would like to **thank:**

Mark Woodward ((WOODY)).

My brother's best friend.

Smiles company entrusts. x

I would like to **thank:**

Uncle Roger Windebank Woof. X

I would like to **thank:**

Phillip Rose - my old friend Comprehensive Mayfield School Portsmouth. He looked after me like big brother.

We had great times Fishing off Southseas Pier. X

I would like to **thank:**

Sandy - step mum - Children: Mandy Chambers Harry/ Jessica.

Simon her Son. Decent people. x

I would like to **thank:**

Debbie The post office lady. Park Parade Shopping Centre. x

I would like to **thank:**

All my **Kick starter Sponsors** - from book 1.

Especially, Edwina Parker X

Edwina gifted me £50 with (Thank you - card) - my first book - The Plain Truth - 3 books she requested I sent. Very kind Spirit. Good friend.

Especially, Mel Croucher. Thank you. x

Mel's belief in me ((backing me)) off his own back.

Especially, Lynden Stowe. Lynden from Gloucestershire sponsor/owner of publishing company - was willing publish my first book. Lynden offered me - a gift - a thank you me my first book. Thank you friend Lynden. x

Especially, Oliver Millen, Sponsor. Thank you. x

I would like to **thank:**

My Physio Therapist, Nurse **Martha.**

I would like to **thank:**

Mark - of Farnborough Surrey, a contractor working on behalf of Waverley B.C. who fitted my ((Storage Heaters)) in my new maisonette - all 5 Dimplex economy 7 heaters.

Mark took away my old heaters, no matter of the extra work involved ((he cared enough)), took them off my hands. So relieved.

Thank you - so much Mark. x

I would like to **thank:**

More Importantly I'd like deep thank you my Readers, whoever Reads Free footed. x

I would like to **thank:**

My Book Publisher: Tricorn Books. **Gail Baird** and **Dan Bernard.**

Patience, effort, Copy editing/Proof reading my books word for word - Grammar, Punctuation, Spell - Checked. 1stly by me then Gail.

I use a free software program, I write my Manuscripts laid out Saved. The ((spell checker)), checks words by automatic process mainly in American English only, with odd algorithms built In - so Apologies.

My words 'underline Red' whenever my Manuscripts Spellings, dissatisfy Software's Program I use formatted, even when many many times correct by Oxford English Dictionary.

Looking tidy I use an American 'Z' replaces an English 'S' or I use one 'L' instead '2 L's' avoiding Red lines looks tidier, as I Write - so go with my lesser preferences, niggles benefit with hindrance either way. So hey, perfections looked for, comes with reasons. My Apologies.

Checking mountainous, rechecking before releases my worked Manuscripts - goes without me saying - thank you so much - Gail Tricorn Books.

No - one single man - believes 'One book' occupying lonely library bookshelf sleeps cost unseen effort.

On the Publishing team is Dan Bernard. Strength, makes things look easy hidden hard-work temperament - gives cause he Wants to, not cause he has to. A Glow handshake about Dan encourages you. You may Walk 1,000 miles ahead Exceed yourself terrain Mistakes Welcome Landscape - Dan is Fair.

Accompanied Dan's presence, Designs Front Cover layout, Back Cover, discuss Colour scheme, Lettering, Size, mix match Ideas, Pictures, Photos, Designs Fab enough. Forward a bit back a bit. Stop just like That.

Run high feelings (no need) - Gail and Dan unhurried, no ending in sight Care.

I Recommend Tricorn Books - Personal at Home Winter log Country pub kinda love - just be Yourself.

Gail Baird, Dan Bernard - Sincere thank you long hours, days and nights you pour shaping - my book's life.

Grateful. Less is more. Gail & Dan. Godspeed. xx

I would like to **thank:**

Bill Furlong. ((Author))

Bill lovely man. Bill suffers struggles same as me with Autism/A.S. and Bill has a Story to tell.

If you are looking to take your Reading further, then do

buy Bill's Books:

Book 1: **Where there's a Bill there's a Way.**

Book 2: **Bill's Way.**

Perspective of Autism told by another, thus educating you, a message you may pass on helping others ignorance or little knowledge. Thank you. Simon x

I would like to **thank:**

The Lord Mayor of Portsmouth - (at the time).

Ms Lynne Stagg. x

I would like to **thank:**

Government/Political figures. x

I would like to **thank:**

Imelda, Personal Adviser at Guildford Job Centre plus. X

Sally, Personal Adviser at Guildford Job Centre plus. X

Sally's help has been indispensable to my performance as I begun moulding my way, a sensible way forward. She works with me every step way, improving my chances to stand on my own two feet, my long term plan. X

I would like to **thank:**

Religious Faith. x

I would like to **thank:**

The Sun Inn Village Pub of Surrey Hills. Village Locals. x

I would like to **thank:**

My fellow Bell-ringers St Mary's and All Saints Church.

Guy Tower master, Joshua Campanology Teacher. x

My - **forgot** to **mention list:**

From ((Book 1 Plain Truth)) **Thank you List:**

1. **Sal Evans.**

From Wolverhampton Birmingham. A very good friend Social

media. x

2. **Sara Jane Davies.**

Sally's Cousin from Wolverhampton. friend. x

3. **Sarah Weeks.**

My loved friend from Sharps Copse Junior School. A.k.a. Sarah Bellinger today. Sarah my long standing friend and social media computer kind nature, strong compassionate. x

4. **Mohamed Elbadri.**

Simon's Dentist Clarendon Rd. Southsea. Portsmouth. Thank you Mo. x

Also Mohamed's downstairs Receptionist, **Donna.** Gowers Dentist. x

5. **Dr Rodin.**

Simon's Doctor friend helped Simon's Diagnosis. St James Hospital Originally.

Own practice: Acorn Lodge. Wymering Portsmouth. x

6. **My C.P.N** Doctor person. **Mick Haley.**

The man who made my recognized Diagnosis at Mill House Hostel Portsmouth. x

Notes from the **Author:**

This Book was written by Simon. R. Newell of his own volition.

Information in this book, will and may change through history. I hope when you read my book, new policies and old, moaned or disagreed with. In fashion, out fashion changes - for better or worse, after my publication - can only mean you wonder why I'd argue out something now apparently agreed/ disagreed. Truth of today's New position augmented alterations.

Staying me I am unchanged long. Only alter egos and why when others change to suit higher credibility In fashion today, isn't so much them. You temporarily all of a sudden remember this is me - ((not changed not changing)).

So do bear in mind dates of publication, minus near two years, the book took turning around writing updating forever shaping Unchanged status, requires Change till it's Right, sat Happy - isn't everyone's status.

With 5 - (Copy edits and Proof reads) each taking me - 3 with 5 months per circular edit. Then remember where possible people's attitudes are changing, evolving back and fourth. I can't change re edit my argument simply cause I gave you a ((one take)) on my 1st Unchanged position, of many positions unchanged coming In.

Fore I'd be writing Encyclopedias here for years to come and you don't want that right? Cause I'm not graced such time. I condensed my book as Is and so look at its size.

Should nothing Change in terms of Policy, towards your Take on Things - then sudden Change - Waters you belief, so only it claims 'conveniences' of help for us in short spells, they claim was always there, till like the Tide no One notices - help was Illusive.

Ways - the better Ways people Act towards you, the way I'd hope. Then enjoy, Read, accept, these views from me ((a Take I gave)) - are 'One Take'. We keep fighting harder turn around something, that mustn't be Fought.

I walks alone. Follow. :-)

Simon Newell
36 Gregs Meadow
Dunsfold
Godalming
Surrey
GU8 4ND

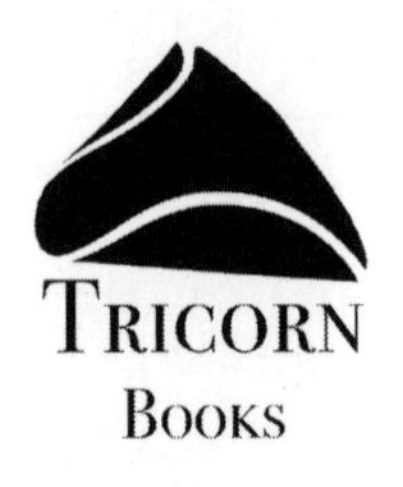